Playing in the Dirt

The key to sustainable health

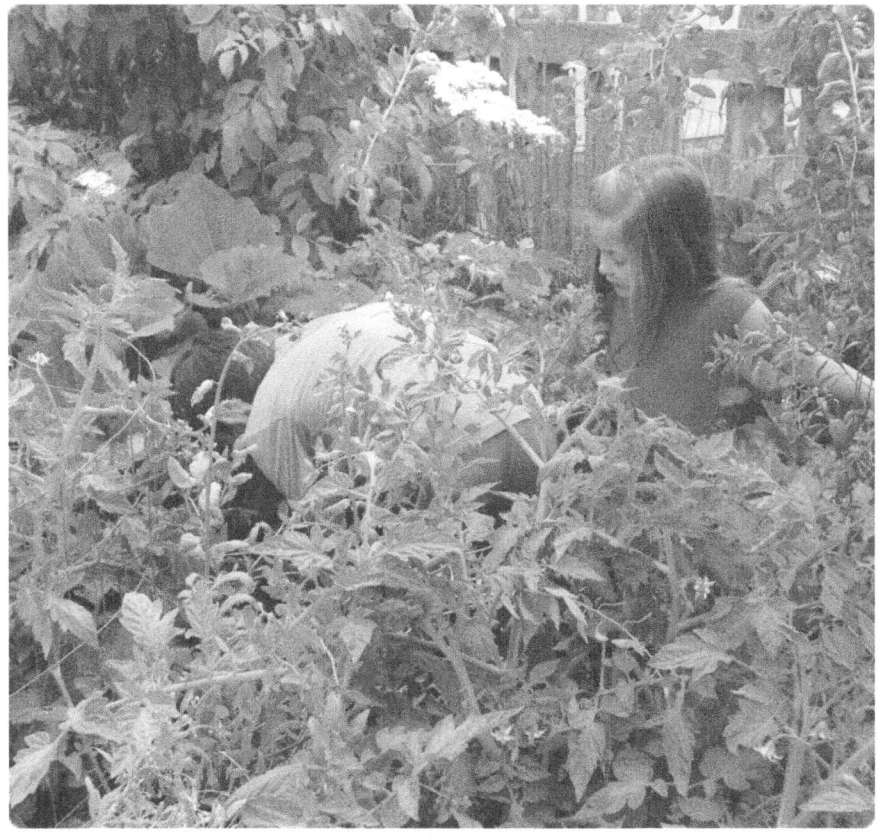

Benjamin Page D.C.

You are built to be healthy.	6
Who are you?	9
We are an integral part of a bigger ecosystem.	14
The consequence of humans abandoning their responsibility	16
Planet Earth is not doing so well.	25
We are an integral part of the ecosystem called Planet Earth.	27
Provide proper nutrition without worry.	33
Early years and nutrition	36
Nutrition as an adult	41
The beauty and health-giving capacity of our home	53
Earth and its beauty	53
Gardening and movement	57
Soil, the natural de-stressor	62
Playing in the dirt and community	64
Soil—fresh, clean, pleasant, and medicinal!	69
Humans and soil	74
Gut bacteria and our well-being	89
The garden and meditation	95
In the zone	97
Finding the time in this modern world	106
A lifestyle – gardening and meditation	109
Mindfulness in the garden	118
Earth and our natural electrical state!	127
My escape	127
Nature wants to help!	131

Earthing!	135
Inflammation is the underlying cause of most chronic illnesses.	137
The earth literally grounds us.	143
Playing in the dirt!	151
Acknowledgments	166
About the author	168

You are built to be healthy.

What is my potential as a human being? What is your potential as a human being? What are we capable of as human beings? According to David Goggins, a former Navy SEAL who has accomplished physical feats that most would think impossible, believes that most people don't even reach 40 percent of their potential capacity as human beings. I couldn't agree more. Not only do most people not even reach 40 percent of their potential as human beings, they pretty much give up on their most important asset—their health!

Why would I call health one of our most important assets? Try doing anything well when you don't feel your best. You might not even be sick, just down and out due to lack of sleep. If you aren't feeling well, if you're not healthy, you can't help yourself, and you surely can't help others.

For some odd reason, we are never taught to invest in our most important assets. Most people finish school not knowing anything about how to invest their time, and their earnings, much less in their health. Why is that? While that is a whole book in and of itself, *Playing in the Dirt* is about one course of action that we can all take to invest in our most important asset—our health.

We have been taught to take medication or supplements or go to therapy for pretty much everything. Modern medicine encourages us to leave our health in the trust of other people and in pharmaceuticals rather than to implement new or improve old lifestyles and trust in our own potential to heal. When something does not feel right, we go to the doctor and get medication or get referred to a therapist to "feel better." Yes, a lot of times we do start to "feel better." Does that mean we are healthier? In most cases, the answer is, unfortunately, no. We then have to continue to return to the doctor so we can get tests done to make sure everything looks great on paper and to make sure everything is staying in between the "normal ranges" on blood tests and other types of panels that are used to measure health in the modern medical paradigm. We are all so different and distinct in our own special ways that we shouldn't be bunched together into certain ranges called "normal" just because on paper 95 percent of people fall into that range. We take blood or other types of bodily fluids at one moment in time and base our overall health on those numbers taken at one precise moment in time. That is not how health should be measured.

I am the perfect example. I have a normal pulse of about 45. I go to the doctor and they check my pulse. When they see that it is not in between the normal ranges of 60 to 90, their first thought is that something must be wrong with me.

We might look normal on the outside and on paper, but what about on the inside? Well, that is a whole different story. Inside, our body is screaming for help. It is trying to let you know what it needs, but medication dulls out that scream. Then we go on with our daily activities worse off than before, until the inevitable happens—the crisis. There's the rush to the hospital, wondering what went wrong. I was taking the right amount of the medication I was prescribed, so why is my body shutting down?

This is all too common in today's world. If you haven't gone through it, I'm pretty sure you know someone who has. It doesn't have to be like that. It shouldn't be like that! We shouldn't live the first twenty-five years ignoring what our bodies need to be healthy, causing stress that will eventually create a symptom; spend the next twenty-five years with symptoms and pain, taking over-the-counter medication to be able to function; and then spend the next twenty-five years with a diagnosed disease where we are on prescribed medication until we die of the same disease we were diagnosed with all those years earlier. That's not to mention all the medication that must be taken to counteract the side effects of the prescribed medication and the loss of quality of life such side effects bring.

There are ways to invest in our most important asset, and this book details one of those ways. You have so much potential! Your health can improve by leaps and bounds when you make the conscious decision to change lifestyles. One of those lifestyles is PLAYING IN THE DIRT!

Who are you?

I wrote an article a while back to help people at a subconscious level to reprogram their thinking of who they are. I suggested repeating a phrase over and over again during a specific time of the day, every day. That phrase was, "I am an ecosystem of trillions of cells programmed for health." What does that mean? Well, let's dive into that a little.

First, what is an ecosystem? An ecosystem is a biological community of interacting organisms and their physical environment. It is a complex network of interconnected systems. That is what we are—a community of cells that interacts with each other all day, every day. They work together, but what are they working toward?

Our cells are constantly working toward health. They are constantly working to build a healthy environment for themselves. This ecosystem is very complex. It's so complex that we will never fully understand it, which is not a bad thing at all. We don't need to fully understand it to be as healthy as possible.

In an ecosystem, every system is interconnected. No single system works alone; they all work together. If one is not functioning correctly, that means others will also not be able to function correctly.

When we don't feel "right," we experience pain or some other type of symptom. It is never just one thing that caused it. I can't tell you what specifically caused that pain in your neck because it is many things, probably thousands of things, over many years. No one can give you a specific answer. That is why looking for the cure really never works. But what does work is building healthy lifestyles.

We are made up of trillions of cells, and I'm glad those cells came together to make the shape we are—that of a human being—because it is a nice shape!

And we are programmed for health. You, yes you, were born with all the internal programming for health. Your body constantly seeks health at all times. There is not a minute of your life where your body is not working toward it.

At the heart of it, we are more than 100 percent capable of living a wonderful life of health because that is what our bodies constantly work toward.

Well, that sounds easy, and for the most part, it is. All we have to do is choose to live lifestyles that are congruent with what our cells require so that they can constantly do what they do—work toward health.

Before we go any further, I want to stop and write just a little about lifestyles and why we need to look at our health in terms of lifestyles. Also, I want to write about why it can be difficult to integrate some healthy lifestyle choices into our lives.

A lifestyle is the way in which a person lives. This is not done once or even twice–this is something that becomes part of us. It is done year after year. It becomes an integral part of our lives, of who we are. Our health is a process, and we have to enjoy the process because the process is all we have. There is no end or finish line, there is only a lifestyle.

If we want to improve or implement new lifestyles, we often have to change. This change for many of us can be difficult, and for that simple reason, it usually will not last long. This is true even if the change is for our own good. Some choices will be more difficult than others. There are many factors to this, but it all comes back to our belief systems. Our belief systems are at the core of everything because our thoughts and actions are based on what we believe and, more importantly, what we feel deep down.

At first as we incorporate a new or better lifestyle, it may be hard. Why? Because deep down we still don't know, we still don't feel, that it is a healthy lifestyle. We haven't changed that belief system. One of the most common healthy lifestyles that doesn't last long is the incorporation of more movement. Deep down we see it—and most importantly, we feel it—as hard and painful and tiring.

How long do you think you will last doing something that you think is hard, painful, and just outright tiring? Not too long. That is why the majority of us only reach 40 percent of our potential. We have so much more to give, and if we will just suffer good through those first difficult times and change the belief system to beautiful instead of hard, joyful instead of painful, and completely fulfilling and invigorating from outright tiring, we will wake up every day with not only the desire to move more, but we will have already put it on our schedule for the day.

If we want a long-lasting change in a lifestyle choice, we have to go all the way to the core and change our belief systems—we have to feel it. This is the part that depends on us and many times can cause suffering. We must embrace that suffering, knowing we will grow and be better because of it, and soon enough, the suffering will turn to joy. The hard part is learning that short-term suffering will evolve into long-lasting joy and that it is nothing compared to what each and every one of our cells have to do every day. If we consciously choose lifestyles where we provide all necessary nutrients and avoid all pollutants, our cells will do the rest.

In today's world, that can be easier said than done. But it is possible if we change our belief systems. One of those important belief systems is the phrase I stated earlier: "I am an ecosystem of trillions of cells programmed for health."

You are an ecosystem of trillions of cells programmed for health!

We are an integral part of a bigger ecosystem.

Have you ever thought about how we fit into this whole crazy ball of water and dirt called Planet Earth?

Do we rule over it? Are we its master? Do we control it?

Just like us, Planet Earth is a biological community of interacting organisms within a physical environment. It is a very complex network of interconnected systems, and we are an integral part of that complex network. We have our job, just like each cell in our body has its job. If that cell in our body can't do its job correctly—in other words, if that cell must adapt due to an unhealthy environment in which we place it—that will cause a chain of events where many systems won't be able to function properly. That one cell has a very important job, which has many effects on the systems throughout our ecosystem.

Just like that one cell, we also have an important job to do in the ecosystem called Planet Earth. I can promise you that the job is not to control it. We are not the masters of nature. Our job is to learn from nature; we are the students and must work with nature, side-by-side.

The consequence of humans abandoning their responsibility

Humans throughout history have always looked to have control; seeking to control nature is no exception. For centuries now, humans have tried to manipulate the natural healthy ways that nature maintains itself. Of course, this was, and almost always is, for the sake of helping humanity. Somehow, humanity thinks the only way to feed the world is to do it in ways that go completely against nature. It works for a while, but eventually, nature wins. Nature inevitably always ends up winning.

When humans started to plant their own gardens, they had ways to keep the soil somewhat fertile on a small scale. To do this, every year they had to till the ground, disrupting the web of life that is beneath our feet. It works, but it is very labor-intensive and a constant uphill battle to keep the garden soil fertile enough to grow nutrient-dense vegetables.

I have beautiful memories of a garden when I was a young kid. I am not going to lie. At that age, they weren't that beautiful. As a kid, I had more important things to do than play in the dirt gardening. There were toy tractors and Legos. I had other kids to play sports with, too. We loved to run, jump, and do all those things that kids love to do! There was just too much to do and gardening didn't fit in the busy schedule of a kid. To help me understand that the garden was pretty important, my parents gave me the privilege of putting gardening on my schedule, sometimes without me even knowing.

After school and during summer break, I had the great opportunity to weed a row of vegetables. This wasn't just any type of row—it was long. For a kid, it felt like a couple of miles. I wish I knew the exact length now so that I could laugh at what I thought was just too much!

If I remember correctly, my brothers, sisters, and I had to weed a row a day to keep the weeds at bay. This was a lot of work for a little kid, but I did it. And I tried to make the best of it, too. For example, I would always choose a row of tall corn so I could pretend I was in a jungle.

Nowadays, I look back and feel grateful for those moments. They made me who I am and also taught me important lessons about food, life, and work.

Weeding wasn't our only fun time in the garden. We also had to cut back the plant growth before winter settled in. We'd pull all the old plants out or just cut them down to the ground and let them decompose over the winter.

In the spring, I remember on various occasions when we would wake early, pack the shovels into the back of the pickup, and drive a couple of blocks to my dad's friend who had horses. My dad would back the truck up to the horse stalls and we'd scoop out all the horse manure, flinging it into the bed of the truck. Back home, we'd shovel the horse manure over the garden and my dad would rototill the decomposing material from last year along with the horse manure into the dirt.

We waited a couple weeks to let everything decompose. Then once the soil was ready, we would plant the seeds.

Planting has to be one of the best times I had in the garden. I remember many rows of sweet corn—again, miles-long to the seven-year-old me!— where about every six inches someone with a shovel would open a gap in the freshly rototilled ground and someone else would drop in two or three seeds. We'd then sow the seeds for string beans, onion bulbs, tomatoes, lettuce, radishes, carrots, spinach, beets, peas, Swiss chard, cucumbers, zucchini, winter squash, and peppers. I think that covers most of it.

For us to keep the garden soil somewhat fertile—I say fertile because it is very difficult to keep the soil alive when you are tilling it every year—we had to constantly add new nutrients through external inputs, like bringing in horse manure and tilling in the old decomposing organic material from last year's garden. On a small scale, like backyard and front yard gardens, this is possible, and we can keep the soil somewhat fertile and grow nutrient-dense food.

However, on a large scale, the supposedly only way to feed the world scale, it is a totally different story—and not a good one at all. Since the explosion of mono-crop agriculture, we're starting to see the damage we've done by trying to take control of nature. We're seeing fertile land dying by the acres and topsoil being eroded by the tons.

A couple of hundred years ago here in the United States, it wasn't such a problem because the farmers weren't farming so much land at one time. They didn't have hundred-acre to thousand-acre farms of the same crop.

It truly is mind-blowing, and if you have never seen it, it is hard to believe. While I was attending Palmer College of Chiropractic in Davenport, Iowa, I had a brother who was a student at Iowa State University in Ames. We would travel back and forth to hang out every once in a while. It's about one hundred, eighty miles from Davenport to Ames, and about ninety percent of the drive is cornfields as far as the eye can see. You just have to see it to believe it.

The farmers a couple of hundred years ago would cut down the forests because that was the most fertile land. They would till up the land and plant and plant and plant, year after year, until they wouldn't get a positive yield. Once they didn't get enough crops to make ends meet, they would go purchase or sometimes just find another piece of fertile land, usually having to cut down trees in the process and repeat everything again.

Well, there came a point where a lot of the fertile land was used up. The farmers had to figure out something fast. What they discovered was that with just three nutrients, you can get a plant to grow, flower, and give fruit. Those three nutrients were nitrogen, phosphorus, and potassium. So, if they could somehow obtain these nutrients, they could stay on the same piece of land for longer periods of time. Phosphorus and potassium weren't that hard to find but nitrogen was. The big guano boom happened because of the great quest for more nitrogen. Guano is basically the feces of seabirds and bats. What made guano so sought after was its high content of nitrogen, making it a perfect fertilizer for the overworked soils. This reminds me of *Ace Ventura: When Nature Calls - Alrighty then*!

Sadly, it doesn't get any better from there. We soon entered World War I, and that disaster with all its chemical warfare. Not only did they find ways to manufacture potassium, phosphorus, and nitrogen, the nutrients the plants needed to survive in chemical form (I say survive because the poor plants were definitely not thriving) in a laboratory, but they also found ways to manufacture chemicals in the laboratory that kill bugs and weeds.

These practices only got worse after World War II and the Vietnam War. With all these chemicals sitting around, no longer needed for warfare, what were they going to do with them? Spray them on the crops, of course.

Well great, right? We no longer had to worry about weeding thousands of acres of corn, wheat, or cabbage. Unfortunately, there were plants killed that we didn't want to have died. How did we solve that? The answer again was to go against nature and modify the seeds genetically so they would be resistant to the herbicide and pesticides. There was so much money and time spent trying to fabricate a completely unnatural way to grow our food when all we had to do was follow nature's lead.

The main crop is now so weak due to the lack of soil health and the bombardment of chemicals that the seeds need to be genetically modified. Then the seeds can survive the horrible conditions and in their poor pathetic life produce some very nutrient-poor food—that we eventually consume.

To make things even worse, the strong weeds survive the herbicide and leave seeds. Now, the herbicide won't work; the weed has become immune to it. So, they manufacture a stronger herbicide or apply more of the herbicide. This goes on and on and on. Until what? Good question!

The same thing goes with pesticides. A pesticide kills almost all the insects that destroy so many crops, but the strongest ones survive and reproduce, and now, the pesticide doesn't work anymore. The answer? Manufacture a more potent pesticide or spray more pesticide. What does that do? It kills off all the weaker insects, leaving the stronger ones to reproduce and continue to destroy crops. This happens over, and over, and over until what? Good question!

What have we done? We thought—actually, we were pretty sure—that we could control nature and do what we want with it. We won some battles, but the outcome of this war is definitely not looking too good.

Masanobu Fucuoka, one of my favorite natural farmers, said:

"The reason that man's improved techniques seem to be necessary is that the natural balance has been so badly upset beforehand by those same techniques that the land has become dependent on them."

What about the health of the soil? You can describe it in one word: dead. The soil is dead. There is absolutely nothing good that can survive that onslaught of constant chemicals. Everything that was good in the soil is now long gone.

Now we have a plant that is maintained on life support with chemical fertilizers long enough to provide some fruit. That fruit is sprayed a couple of times with herbicides and pesticides.

The last time that grains are sprayed with an herbicide is before harvest where they spray them with even more herbicide, so it kills the grain making the harvesting process that much easier. The grain gets milled, packaged, and shipped probably thousands of miles, and it lands right in your grocery store. That's where you speed by with your shopping cart and pick out the cheapest thing because you are too busy and tired to worry about something so important as what you are eating and providing your family, and in all honesty, your health.

Planet Earth is not doing so well.

In our ecosystem when one cell is not getting the proper amount of nutrition at the right time, it can't do its job properly.

That sounds incredibly difficult to comprehend. For our cells to do their job properly, they must have the proper amount of nutrition at the right time. How in the world are we supposed to know what each cell requires nutritionally, the amount required, and at what time? The answer is that we don't! And really, we don't need to. All we have to do is eat nutrient-dense food grown in fertile soil without chemicals or raised on food grown in fertile soil, move adequately, talk to ourselves naturally, rest adequately, surround ourselves with people that want the best for us and take care of our spines. If we do those six things, our body will provide those nutrients we give it at the right amount and at the right time. That is our ecosystem beyond beautiful and comprehension! I have another book dedicated to this. Check it out. It's called _The 4 Pillars of Health: Your health and well-being made simple!_

Planet Earth as an ecosystem works the same way as our human body ecosystem. To function at its best, it needs everybody doing their job properly. Every other creature in the world, from the elephant to the worm, knows their job and nothing else, and they do it and do it quite well. However, we as humans are just slightly different from other creatures. We have reason, the ability to think things out and come to a conclusion, and then act on that conclusion. This ability to reason is why we are the dominant species in this ecosystem. But with this ability to reason has come much destruction, and we as a species, as well as nature, have suffered.

Since the Industrial Revolution, Planet Earth's ecosystem has suffered incredibly. We have gone from working with nature to working against nature in most agricultural endeavors. And it isn't just agricultural endeavors that are causing so much havoc to the ecosystem. Since the beginning of time, nature has never been so sick.

It is impossible for us to be healthy if where we live is not healthy. When nature becomes sick over time, we too, as humans, will become sick.

That might sound depressing, and in reality, it is. It is sad that we have allowed it to come to this point. But instead of letting it get you down, it should be a wake-up call to all of us to improve or, if needed, change our unhelpful lifestyles. There are so many things we can do—each and every one of us. We can be the change by first simplifying our own lives. This book will also give you another great way to help heal the Earth so we can also heal. It truly can only be done by all of us, as the famous quote by Margaret Mead states,

"Never doubt that a small group of thoughtful, committed citizens can change the world. Indeed, it is the only thing that ever has."

We are an integral part of the ecosystem called Planet Earth.

The first time I heard the word permaculture was in the early days of iPods and podcasts. I lived about five miles from the Palmer campus and on most days, I rode my bike to class. During summer and spring, it took me about fifteen minutes, giving me half an hour total to listen to whatever. In the winter and fall, it took me about forty-five minutes one way, and that was if the ice on the path didn't slow me down.

At first, I listened to music on my iPod. But I soon realized that I could use that time just a little more intelligently. A new thing had started and a couple of people were talking about it. This new thing was called a podcast where people talked about different topics. The listeners had the ability to choose what they wanted to listen to by subscribing to a podcast that interested them.

Wow, incredible! I didn't have to listen to some talking heads just because they were the only talking heads available.

At school, a couple of my buddies and I were interested in a topic called modern survivalism, and they had mentioned a podcast called *The Survival Podcast* by Jack Spirko.

I subscribed and started downloading all the episodes. At that time, if I remember correctly, he had a total of eight episodes. Today, he has well over two thousand.

I don't remember exactly which episode he introduced permaculture to me, but that one word changed how I see the world completely. Just one word sent me on a journey to figure out how I could grow food in a sustainable manner. Not just sustainable but actually in a way that would improve the soil life of my garden year after year. A term being used now is regenerative agriculture. Regenerative agriculture needs to be used on the mega-farms and in each and every little garden we have in our front and backyards.

This means not only is it important that the ranchers and farmers implement regenerative agriculture but you and I as well.

Today, about 55 percent of the world's population lives in cities. I prefer to call them concrete jungles. In these concrete jungles, most people have lost total contact with nature. Most haven't even touched soil for years. They are constantly on top of some kind of concrete or asphalt. Not only that but there is always a layer of rubber between our feet and the ground, known as shoes.

Nature, to most kids in the cities, is an open area where automatic irrigation and herbicides keep the grass alive and weed-free. That area of grass is maintained by a lawn tractor that comes and cuts it regularly. There also might be some pruned trees scattered around the area, but not too many because then the kids would not be able to play soccer or football. Don't forget the play area with all its plastic and metal parts and the ground below covered in either sand or recycled tires.

Most adults will sit at a table and watch their kids and then walk around on the concrete walkways, avoiding the grass.

With the majority of people almost completely disconnected from nature, it makes sense that we would not care too much about it. It is out of sight, out of mind.

What happens when we forget about nature? Our health suffers because we are interrelated. We can't hope to be healthy without her in our lives. She does not need us, but we need her. That doesn't mean we have to live out in the woods to be healthy. I do recommend getting out into nature as much as possible, but for many, that is just not possible. What it does mean is that we need to work with her. How does a city dweller do that? One way is by buying food produced by local farmers and ranchers that are working with nature. It is a win-win situation. We can help regenerate our soil and at the same time, nourish our ecosystems. There are also many other ways that a city dweller can work with nature.

This book is not about how, but about why we need to be connected to the Earth, to nature. However, this is just the beginning of our journey together. I will continue to write and create videos on how we can reconnect ourselves.

My hope is that the information you will receive in the following pages will give you a hunger to return to your roots, the desire to return to nature and to come up with new ideas of how to do it. Even more importantly, I hope you share those ideas so we can all become healthier people because deep down that is what we want: to be healthy and happy. Returning to the earth is the fastest, cheapest, and easiest way to do it.

Let's get into why we must return to nature so together we can come up with how to do it! This is going to be great!

Provide proper nutrition without worry.

Most people go back to their roots—or in other words, they begin to garden—because of the food. They don't truly understand why it is so important to reconnect themselves to the earth. They are either tired of the industrial food system that is slowly poisoning them and decide to take things into their own hands, or they just want a simpler life. Either way, they begin to play in the dirt and provide not just proper nutrition but also what their bodies truly require and deserve to be able to take full advantage of what life has to offer. Nutrient-dense food is one of the many benefits we receive while playing in the dirt!

Nutrition has become a multibillion-dollar industry, and on many occasions, I have wondered why. Not only do people spend hundreds of dollars on ways to supply nutrition to our deprived bodies through supplements and other drinks, teas, and food products, but also the amount of money spent on research to find out how much of a macro or micronutrient is needed for highest performance is mind-boggling. These nutrients, mostly vitamins and minerals, are studied just like disease is—in isolation.

They don't take into account how one nutrient will affect how the body will use other nutrients. As an ecosystem, we are constantly working together and never working separately.

To be completely honest, we will never know exactly what the body needs in the amount necessary at the precise moment. Our ecosystem is just too complex. There is a solution, though, and it is much easier than worrying about giving your body enough of the one or two nutrients that a blood test showed that you were a little below or above average in. And most of these tests only check for macronutrients. There are also many micronutrients that we must provide our ecosystem of cells with to be well and healthy.

It's a battle that we just can't win. We have to let go of the thinking that through testing we can know exactly what nutrition our body needs and give the body only that. Nutritionally, we will just never know exactly.

It sounds depressing, but it is actually the opposite. It should be a relief, one less worry in a life already jam-packed with activities. We only have a certain amount of energy that is provided for decision-making every day, and once that energy is used up, most decisions are bad or just not made at all. The decisions needlessly made on nutrition can free up so much of that decision-making energy. And for those that don't understand the importance of nutrition, it is the same. By doing one thing, the whole debate over nutrition or the lack of knowledge of nutrition becomes unnecessary.

That one thing is to grow your own food, and what you can't grow, get it as local as possible from farmers you can trust. It sounds daunting and difficult, but once you get some systems in place, it becomes quite simple and more economical. Of course, playing in the dirt can be hard and frustrating at times, but in its entirety, with systems in place, it becomes simple and very enjoyable.

There are two times in my life that I remember clearly when I didn't worry about nutrition at all. One was when I was a kid. Without me knowing, I was getting pretty good nutrition. The other was when I was an adult and I consciously knew what I was consuming. Unfortunately, those times haven't lasted forever, and sometimes, I still worry if I am giving my body the nutrition it requires. I don't have all the systems in place that make my eating habits worry-free.

At the same time, what we look for is the best possible decision in the environment in which we put ourselves. For example, at parties there are usually consumable products offered; if we have the proper systems in place, we can have nutritious food with us or decide to fast and not eat anything that will slowly poison us. If we make the decision to eat, it is important to let it go and not stress over what we just ate. That surely doesn't help either. We are not perfect; we are only trying, and as trying implies we will fail sometimes. It is part of life and it is how we learn and grow.

Early years and nutrition

Before I was nine years old, I had no idea what nutrition was. I ate what my parents gave me. From what I know now, and what I remember from then, it was in a manner that was in harmony with what my body required and deserved. Just imagine a nine-year-old being asked what their favorite food is and hearing, "Smashed potatoes and smashed squash, all mixed together with salt, butter, vinegar, and pepper." Yup, that was me. I have always loved that stuff. Was it easy for my parents and us kids? No. But it was simple.

Being on my hands and knees as a kid, pulling weeds out of the many rows of corn, peas, and green beans was not easy, but eating them did make my nutrition simple. Waking up early to feed the chickens and sneakily fitting myself in the little doorway of the coop, hoping the rooster didn't see me and charge at me while I grabbed some eggs, was not easy. But eating that egg after my mom cooked it made my nutrition simple.

Watching my grandfather butcher and clean a chicken, then my mother taking that chicken and cooking it was not easy for them, but it made my nutrition simple. My brother milking the goat early every morning wasn't easy for him, and when I would help my mom make butter and cheese from the cream of the milk, that was also not easy. But using that butter to fry an egg made my nutrition simple. Sprinkling some salt on the goat cheese and eating it made my nutrition simple. Harvesting plums, apples, and peaches off of the trees in our backyard was not easy but it sure made my nutrition simple.

At the time, I didn't understand anything about nutrition. I just ate what there was, and fortunately, what was available was nutrient-dense.

Was it easy? No. But what good comes out of easy? Was it simple? Yes. I ate nutrient-dense food, and my body did the rest. I provided what my body needed, and it used the food at the right time and in the proper amount, or stored it for later use. There was absolutely no worry.

Those early years were just what my little developing body needed. There was lots of time outside in the sun playing in the dirt and growing nutrient-dense food in fertile soil without chemicals. I remember more fun and games than the work outside, but that does not mean we didn't work a lot and that it wasn't difficult for my parents. They had their work for sure, and we helped out as much as we could.

Those rows and rows and rows of corn had to be harvested eventually, and when they were, not only did we get the privilege of eating incredibly clean, nutrient-dense sweet corn, but we also got the opportunity to blanch a lot of corn and then cut the kernels off the cobs and place them in Ziploc bags to store and eat later. My mom would cut the corn off in strips, and oh, how I loved grabbing those strips of sweet corn and gobbling them up.

I heard on many occasions, "Ben, stop eating the corn and put it in the bags." My job was to place the freshly-cut corn into Ziploc bags that would then go into the huge freezer we had out in the garage for later use. We had corn from the garden pretty much all year long.

Then came the peas. With rows of peas ready to be picked, we all got to it. We picked buckets of them. We couldn't eat them all when they were just picked, and that wasn't the plan anyway. My parents planted a lot of corn, peas, and green beans knowing that the majority of these vegetables were going to be preserved for later use. That didn't stop me from eating a lot of sweet peas, though. First, I would take the peas out of the pods, and then the peas were supposed to go into a big bowl. But again, over and over, I would hear, "Ben, stop eating the peas." I would open the pod and see those sweet peas, and they were just too tempting. Instead of the bowl, they went straight into my mouth. I can taste the explosion of sweet flavor in my mouth to this day.

Then the unforgettable and still-to-this-day favorite vegetable that came straight out of the garden: green beans. Man, how I enjoyed—and still enjoy—green beans. Getting a bucket and a row to myself, I would begin to pick all the ripe green beans until my bucket was full—of course, eating as I went. What we didn't eat fresh got blanched and prepared to freeze. Slightly boiled green beans with salt on top—not much better than that! Life was good, really good (for those that have watched the movie *Nacho Libre,* ha-ha-ha).

It wasn't just the abundance of food found in the garden that provided my little body the proper nutrition in the right amount at the right time, either. Close to home there was a man-made lake always stocked with fish, mostly trout. My older brother loved fishing, and I tagged along on occasion.

We would usually catch a couple fish, gut and clean them, and then eat them fresh or place them in the huge freezer out in the garage for future protein and fats so important to our nutrition.

From fresh eggs, chicken, fish, goat milk and goat cheese, to corn, squash, green beans, peas, tomatoes, onions, and many other vegetables, to peaches, apples, and plums, I had a variety of nutrition right in front of me and didn't even know it. I look back at those years and don't have one bad memory. I am sure at that age that I complained about the work, but I did it and am glad that I had the opportunity. I learned the importance of work at a very young age by working in the garden. I am beyond grateful to my parents for giving me that opportunity to work—I mean play—and for the abundance of nutrition that my developing body needed in those times that were so important to overall health.

Nutrition as an adult

At nine years old, we moved to Las Vegas, a city in the desert. My parents tried to plant a garden in that summer heat with little rainfall, but it was difficult. I remember them trying tomatoes and peppers. As time went on, I eventually finished high school, joined the Marine Corps, and went through Marine Corps basic training, served a religious mission in Puebla, Mexico, went to college, and worked in all sorts of construction jobs.

During those years of construction, in the morning and college in the evening, I went on a trip to Argentina with my grandma. There, one of my mom's cousins introduced me to my future wife. We would eventually get married and have two awesome kids..

After completing my undergraduate work, I applied to Palmer College of Chiropractic in Davenport, Iowa, and was accepted. We packed up all we had into a small trailer and the bed of our 2005 GMC Canyon and made the two-day trip to Davenport to start my studies to become a chiropractic physician. As you will see in a future chapter, it was while I was studying at Palmer College of Chiropractic that I slowly began to return to my roots and play in the dirt again.

Palmer is where I got an introduction to nutrition and its importance in our health. However, it was after Palmer when I was working as a chiropractic physician that my own desire to understand nutrition really took shape. I began to study on my own about nutrition and, most importantly, the best methods on how to provide our bodies with proper nutrition.

While working as a chiropractic physician, I had a small garden. And since I was only able to grow a small percentage of our food, my wife and I decided we would spend less on some things to be able to spend a little more on the food we could trust to be nutrient-dense. In that moment in my life, I started to feel that we were building a pretty neat system where we were eating healthy. In other words, we were providing our ecosystem of cells what they required and deserved.

Through all this time, my parents had pretty much retired and moved back to the town where I had lived the first nine years of my life.

I started to realize that the job I was in was putting a lot of physical stress on my joints and that in the long run would cause unnecessary pain and suffering if I continued the way I was working.

Through a lot of discussions over yerba mate, we finally came to the decision to leave where I was working and pursue a slightly different path. This was not an easy decision with a family to support. I would work as a chiropractic physician during the afternoon and in the mornings, work as a farmer raising chickens on pasture for meat. This was for two reasons: (1) to take some of the physical stress off my joints due to the repetitive movement against the weight that chiropractic cause on the physician, and (2) to supply my family first, and then patients, with a meat that is raised properly and nutrient-dense. I wrote about the chicken farm in my first book *The 4 Pillars of Health: Your Health and Well-being Made Simple*.

To be able to accomplish these goals, we needed some land, a place to properly raise chickens. Well, that took us back to my birthplace, that place of so many good memories.

Since we didn't have a lot of money, we sold the majority of the items we owned. I even sold my 1995 red Jeep Wrangler. That wasn't easy, but it was necessary for the change in our lives. We packed up what was left and went and lived with my parents while I started this new venture with my family.

I am not going to lie. It was hard on me mentally. I thought and said to myself probably thousands of times, "You have a family and you are moving into your parents' house." I definitely did not feel like a good parent or husband doing this, which didn't help my internal dialogue that became pretty mean. However, I tried to stay optimistic by planning on everything working out for the best in many ways, which included not only the relief of the physical stress that a high-volume chiropractic clinic brings but also the other stresses that plague modern living today.

Besides the mental anguish I put myself through, there was a lot of good that came out of that experience of farming and chiropractic. To tell you the truth, this book would never have happened if it wasn't for the decision we made that day in Las Vegas while drinking mate outside with our feet in the little inflatable pool we had for our kids. I still remember it as if it was yesterday. My wife was in black-and-pink shorts and a black tank top because she had been in the pool with the kids. Her feet were against the pool wall, pretty much tucked-in like a ball, and I was in my work clothes with my pants rolled up and my feet dangling in the water. We both looked at each other and said, "Well, let's do it." That set this all into motion, and here I am today writing these words.

It isn't just this book though; the period of time when we returned to that little town in southern Utah was a time in my life where my nutrition again was not a question or a worry.

It wasn't perfect or even ideal, as you will see, but it was one less worry. We moved at the end of summer. My parents were harvesting a lot from their garden and eating foods mostly from the garden. We got there just in time to help out. Before we headed out, I had ordered my first fifty Cornish Cross chicks that were going to be delivered the same week we got there. Cornish Cross chickens are the classic bird used for meat. They are the cutest little yellow puffballs out there.

My kids were super excited when I got the call from the post office letting me know they had arrived. I had prepared everything the day before. I was using two big plastic storage bins filled with pine shavings for bedding as a starter pen. The smell was wonderful. There was a long feeder in one bin and a round feeder in the other. Both bins both had round waterers. Each bin also had its own heat lamp. The bins were kept inside the house. Yup, the chicks for the first two weeks lived with us inside the house. You have to remember I was learning; this was all new to me. I would add fresh pine shavings every day and every week change it completely, throwing all the pine shavings into the compost bin. That kept the smell nice and clean.

While taking care of fifty chicks, I was also preparing a bigger chicken coop that would hold them until they were about a month old. I also had to complete another big coop that would hold them during their last month. At the same time, I was getting my little practice up and going. The local dentist allowed me to use a small room in his office to start and treat patients in the afternoon when he had finished for the day. I also had to learn how to build a webpage and start a podcast about health and gardening: two things I knew absolutely nothing about. Fun times! Now with over two hundred episodes, I have a little more experience. If you like, check it out: _The Wellness Farmer Podcast_.

In between all those fun times, I was also able to play in the dirt, helping my parents harvest from their two gardens. What an abundance they had that summer and fall!

There were moments that were truly beautiful—moments that brought me back to when I was a kid. My two kids, my grandma Lita, and my mom and dad picked peas from the backyard garden.

Then we would sit around a table outside, usually under a tree, and separate the peas from the pods. This time it was me telling my two kids, "Matías, Verena, the peas go into the bowl." They opened up the pods and more often than not the peas went into their mouths instead of the bowl, just like I did over twenty years before.

Again, just like when I was a kid, we were eating from the garden. Not everything, but a good amount. I was able to play in the dirt with my kids while we picked green beans and peas. My kids, just like me, loved green beans, but they added a little butter instead of just salt. They absolutely loved the sweet corn and usually asked for corn on the cob first thing before eating anything else. Among the green beans and peas and corn, there was zucchini, tomatoes, peppers, carrots, potatoes, cilantro, and many different types of lettuce among other nutrient-dense foods.

Many times, my wife asked me to go dig up potatoes, cut some zucchini, or cut some lettuce for dinner that same night. It was garden-to-plate. Just beautiful! It felt so simple. I did not say easy; I said simple. Instead of thinking about my nutrition, I was able to enjoy the beauty of what fertile soil brings while sitting around a table with the most important people in my life.

The garden was just one part of the system. There were also raspberries, goji berries (also known as wolfberries), sea buckthorn berries, strawberries, and red and black currants. There were apples, plums, and peaches as well.

Then there were chickens raised in a beautiful manner, where they lived a great life as chickens, sunbathing, scratching, pecking, drinking fresh well water, eating grass and bugs, and their diets supplemented with non-GMO organic feed. They lived practically a stress-free life, protected from predators, and allowed to live as chickens should. My favorite time of every day was in the morning when I would move the chicken coop to fresh green grass. They would go crazy running around looking for bugs and then settle down and start eating fresh blades of grass.

That was not all we ate; we also bought food. We made a monthly trip to a supermarket where we could buy organic meats and other produce. We spent a little more on these foods, but with a lot of food coming from the beautiful healthy soil from where we lived, we didn't have to buy as much.

If you remember, I wrote that I didn't have to worry, but at the same time, it wasn't ideal. I used these words because we had to buy organic produce from the supermarket. It would be even better to get your meats, if you consume them, from a local farmer that you know is raising the animals in the way the animal should naturally live. I will never forget the great quote from Joel Salatin that says:

"Our motto is we respect and honor the pigness of the pig and the chickenness of the chicken. That means not confining them in a house with hundreds of others."

We need to look to ranchers and farmers that understand the role of the animals and allow the animals to accomplish their role, which is very important. Animals can only do that if they are allowed to live the lives they deserve.

The photo on the inside cover is of my kids taking care of their own plants. My son decided he wanted a bell pepper plant, and my daughter decided she wanted a watermelon plant. My son's plant provided the peppers needed for delicious chile relleno on more than one occasion. My son was planting and eating nutrient-dense food grown in fertile soils without chemicals. Just beautiful and all at the age of nine years old.

These two times in my life, one as a child and the second with my children, have truly impacted me. I will never forget that part of my life as a child and how it helped me build a strong, healthy foundation for the future. I hope that my kids will also remember those times when they were also building a healthy foundation.

Food is where nutrition is assimilated. We can take all sorts of supplements and medicines but what the body truly is asking for is nutrient-dense food. That is all it wants and all it needs. What better place to provide your body with just that than through your own garden? By playing in the dirt, we can provide the nutrition required to maintain our ecosystem called the human body.

The garden makes it simple; if it is your garden, it makes it fresher, meaning more nutritious. There is nothing fresher than harvesting from your front or backyard and going straight to the kitchen.

Many of you might live in an area where you have very little land—like me at this moment in my life. I have a very small piece of land that is in-between the street and the sidewalk. That is it—all other plants are in planter boxes. It doesn't matter where you live; even just growing herbs on your windowsill is a great start. It is something.

If you just start, for some odd reason other opportunities will likely arise. Maybe a community garden nearby you will open up or a friend with more land that isn't being used for anything will let you use it. Or, in my case, after weeks of talking with the municipality, they are going to allow me to use some of the land they have in a community garden.

For many, it just won't happen, and when the opportunity is not there, it is important to get to know local farmers and support their efforts by buying from them.

The beauty and health-giving capacity of our home

No, I am not talking about the four walls and a roof that we call home. I am talking about our only home, at least for now—Earth. Just as we take care of the four walls and roof we call home, we should be doing the same thing for our home, Earth. The beauty of it is if we do our part taking care of the earth, what the earth gives back will outweigh by a long shot what we put in.

For most people, the only healthy benefit of planting a garden, or as I like to call it, playing in the dirt, is what I finished discussing: nutrient-dense food. The ability to give your body the nutrition it requires. Growing some of your food—or if you are lucky enough, all of your food—of course is a healthy lifestyle choice. But it isn't just because of the nutrient-dense food grown in that soil that is alive and fertile that makes it a healthy lifestyle choice.

Earth and its beauty

Earth is extraordinarily beautiful. There have been dozens of documentaries just on the different beauties of what Earth has to offer. The natural beauty that surrounds us is why most people go on hikes or camping. They go to take in the natural beauty that surrounds them.

Sometimes they travel large distances just to experience the natural beauty of Earth. It feels great to be able to see it, to breathe it, to touch, and experience it.

The more I study about us as humans, the more I become convinced that the "feeling brain" is what is truly in control. Our feeling brain, or in other words our emotions, are where we truly experience the beauty of what life has to offer. Our thinking brain is there to give suggestions and ideas on how to go about our daily tasks and try and keep us on track, but it is only when we feel something that we will make the proper changes in our life. We can know—and I would even go out on the ledge and say that most of us do know—that planting a garden is a healthy lifestyle choice. But until we feel it, it will either never happen or it won't last past the first season.

Nature is also all about feeling. There is no thinking required to experience the beauty of nature, and that feeling heals us. If you work behind a desk all day, how many times have you left the office and gone outside to just feel the air and the sun hit your skin? It brings life back to feel those things; not think about them but to feel them.

The garden, though not truly natural (I recommend growing food in the most natural of ways by following the example of the expert, Mother Nature herself), is a great way to just feel the beauty of what surrounds us. That beauty can be completely man-made with perfectly squared garden beds and perfectly manicured with everything in its place. That is also beautiful, and just being present in that beauty will heal and strengthen you.

Playing in the dirt takes us outside where we can feel nature, feel the sun's rays. The sun's rays are just as important to us as they are to plants.

Yes, if the plants don't receive the sun's rays, they will not be able to photosynthesize, and they will eventually die. We also need to feel those rays, and gardening (playing in the dirt) gets us outside and under the sun where those rays can do their job. The sun is the best source of vitamin D. When the skin is exposed to sunlight, it makes vitamin D from cholesterol, which is another important nutrient that we must provide our ecosystem of cells.

I have written a lot about how animals that are raised on food that is grown in fertile soil, and vegetables and fruits that are grown in fertile soil, are nutrient-dense and provide us with the tools and building blocks to build a healthy environment inside of us. But that isn't where all nutrition comes from. The beauty of being outside and growing some of our nutrient-dense food helps us obtain other nutrients, like vitamin D, that are so important in maintaining our ecosystem.

As we are outside enjoying the health-providing beauty of nature, either in a manmade garden bed or the wilderness, we are feeling the health-promoting rays of the sun and feeling the beauty around us. This beauty not only heals us but is wonderful for our overall physical and mental well-being. Being in nature and taking her in through our senses has a name. In Japan, it is "Shinrin-yoku" translated as "forest bathing." It is something that physicians in Japan promote to their patients as an antidote to hectic urban life. Today, in English, it has been given the name eco-therapy and has improved the health and well-being of many that practice it. By feeling nature, by being with her, we are stronger and healthier, and only through feeling can we truly act. We must feel, not just know to act for our betterment.

I love using the example of exercise. I imagine the majority of people understand and know we not only should but we must, exercise. We must move to be healthy. Exercise is not just for those that want to improve the appearance of their bodies or improve their performance in sports; it is vital for all of us. But how many of us actually exercise, actually get out and move instead of just sitting comfortably on the couch? If we understand, if we know we need to move more, why aren't we doing it three to five times a week? Because we don't feel it, and until we feel we need to exercise, we won't do it, or at least not in a consistent manner, the way we know we should.

Gardening and movement

Not only does the garden get us outside under the sun but it gets us moving. To garden, we must move and at times even lift objects, dig into the dirt, and maybe even break a sweat. Movement is vitally important to our health and well-being.

Movement can be done in many ways. It doesn't have to only happen at a gym or in some class. A great way to get out there and provide some of the movement our ecosystems require is to prepare a garden bed. I am even talking to those people in the age group that think they are too old. Grabbing a shovel and digging is a great form of exercise; it doesn't matter how slow you do it. As long as we don't put all the weight on our lower backs, it will only do us good to get out and move some dirt. Fertile soil is one of the best weights out there and it is free. There is no need for a membership or a place to store it, it is pretty much all around us.

Some of my best moments of movement are found in the garden or out in nature. Exercise has always been something I've liked to do. Anything physical calls my attention, but those days under the sun with a bottle of water, a sturdy pickax and shovel, and the dirt under my feet have been beautiful full-body workouts. Using a shovel and pickax in their proper form will work the shoulders all the way down to the calves. It is one of the best full-body workouts you can get.

Even if you just want to put a little weight against your bones and muscles, again, the garden can't be beaten. There were many times where all I had was a small garden shovel and some seedlings. There I was, moving just enough fertile soil to plant a seedling into my prepared garden bed. Some of my most memorable moments in the garden are those calm movements with my daughter or my son outside planting with me. Those calm moments of movement are a great way to keep inflammation at bay in our joints. Less inflammation means less pain and the ability to enjoy life just that much easier. The more we move, the better we will be off. The garden gives us a huge range of movements, from rigorous to calm.

Again, if you think you're too old, remember that the best thing you can do to stay young and healthy and starve off atrophy is to go outside and play in the dirt. It's vital to your health.

What's so wonderful about movement, or in other words, exercise, is that it doesn't just improve our physical health; it also improves our emotional health. Movement is a wonderful way to decrease stress.

Stress in all its forms causes havoc. Almost all chronic diseases at their roots see inflammation caused by some type of stress. Movement decreases stress and helps prevent chronic disease, from autoimmune diseases all the way to heart disease. As we work those muscles by moving our joints, we are decreasing overall stress and making life just a little more enjoyable and healthier.

How does this happen? Well, in various ways. First, movement can help relax you. It can also increase self-confidence by showing that you at least have control of one thing—your body. It can also help you sleep better at night. Exercise or movement also brings us into the moment, and we focus on the task-at-hand letting everything else go. This is one of the best ways to reduce stress. Then there is the increased production of endorphins, also known as the feel-good neurotransmitters.

Endorphins inhibit the pain pathways, helping us to feel less pain and a great way to reduce stress.

Another effect of endorphins is they can produce a feeling of euphoria. What in the world is euphoria? It is the experience of pleasure or excitement and intense feelings of well-being and happiness. Yup, that is what exercise will do for you. What better place to do it than in the beautiful, health-giving environment of the garden.

The garden and playing in the dirt don't stop at decreasing physical stress and emotional stress; it also can decrease the stresses of everyday living.

One of the things we pretty much must do every day is to eat a meal that is nutrient-dense, which provides the body with what it needs to keep us healthy. Playing in the dirt, in other words planting a garden, can also reduce the stress about the all-important part of life called eating. We have to eat to sustain life. The garden can provide for that. Eating is a necessity of life, not even taking into account the nutrition it provides.

We all know that life can be stressful, and even more, now that we are living the "modern life." Knowing that you have a garden that is growing something to eat is one less stress. If we are lucky enough, we also grow enough to be stored away for later use, decreasing the stresses of everyday life even more.

One of the potential stresses of everyday life is something that happens to millions around the world: the loss of a job. Imagine you lose your job, but at the same time you know you have a garden at home that is providing nutrient-dense food for yourself and your family, and that last year's garden provided a surplus, and you have it bottled at home, ready to eat. You now can put more of your energy toward finding a new job or starting a new business than worrying and stressing about how in the world you are going to feed your family tomorrow.

Soil, the natural de-stressor

If that wasn't enough, playing in the dirt has another great way of decreasing the amount of stress modern living rests on our shoulders. Fertile soil is alive with billions of microorganisms. Just a handful of fertile soil can have up to fifty billion bacteria. Almost all those bacteria will do us no harm, and a lot of them are there to help us. One example of beneficial bacteria is the now popular bacterium found in fertile soils: Mycobacterium vaccae.

One study performed by Christopher Lowry, a neuroscientist at the University of Bristol, and his team injected Mycobacterium vaccae into mice. The mice were then subjected to a series of stress tests. They found that the mice that were inoculated with the bacteria showed far less stressed behavior than their untreated counterparts. In the inoculated mice, the Mycobacterium vaccae activated groups of neurons in the brain responsible for producing serotonin. Serotonin is known as a neurotransmitter that is a contributor to feelings of well-being and happiness.

By breathing around fertile soil and running our hands through it, we are allowing that beautiful bacterium to enter into our ecosystem and help us naturally produce more serotonin, improving our overall well-being and decreasing our overall stress.

That study centered on just one of the billions of bacteria found in fertile soil. It is amazing how much of an integral part the soil is to who we are and how playing in the dirt can reduce the overall stressful life most of us live today.

Playing in the dirt and community

Yesterday was a beautiful spring day. To take advantage of what nature was offering, I grabbed two lawn chairs and went to the only place where we have some grass, right in between the street and the sidewalk.

Our tiny backyard is all covered with cement, and the only fertile soil we have is located within big planter boxes. Out front, there is an area between the street and the sidewalk divided in two by a walkway that makes its way to the front door. It isn't more than eight feet long and twenty feet wide. In one of the divisions, I have my little front yard garden where I grow food for myself and my family, and unexpectedly, also for the community. For some odd reason, people come by and pick what they want without asking. Once it was my lettuce, another time my Swiss chard, and most recently the butternut squash. On the other side of the walkway, there is a small patch of grass.

On that patch of grass, I set up the two lawn chairs. I heated some water, prepared the mate, went outside, took off my shoes and socks, and planted my bare feet in the grass. Man, it felt great! Next to me was my wife. These moments are unforgettable and priceless. I cherish these opportunities. While chatting with my wife, people passed by, including a man named Hugo. He stopped to say hi and added, "Ben, I have been wanting to ask you a question. I planted some cherry tomatoes and want to know if they are ready to transplant?"

I was really excited—he had planted some seeds!

He explained the situation, and yes, they were ready to be transplanted in their own little pots. He had planted a lot of seeds all together and the majority had germinated and were all very close to each other. I explained what he could do and how he could do it, and then we both said goodbye and he went on his way.

Hugo is a really good guy and is taking care of his wife who is not feeling well. I met Hugo one day while I was out front planting the garden with my daughter. While planting, he passed by. I said, "Hi," and a great conversation evolved. We talked about many things, including a garden and his desire to grow some food. Hugo does have a backyard, so the possibilities were great. Since that conversation, Hugo started his garden and is growing nutrient-dense food for himself and his wife.

The garden is a great place to build community. Through my own, I have been able to get to know many people like Hugo who live in our community. While walking by, they usually ask me what I am doing, and then comes the second question, which is almost always the same: "Don't people come and steal it all?" With that question starts a beautiful conversation where trust and friendship develop.

A community is also a great way to reduce the stresses of life, even more today than ever because of the virtual lives most of us are living. Getting out and just talking to someone in the community is a rare experience, but it shouldn't be. Yes, virtual communities are great, and I have accomplished much with the help from them, but they can't take the place of the people around you.

We are animals (of course, with reason) that not only thrive but require a community to be healthy. Contact with other human beings is vitally important to our emotional and physical health. People who know me might be wondering how I can say something like that, being a person who loves to be alone. Yes, when I am alone I do take full advantage of it; however, there are moments where I yearn to be with others and communicate with them. It is natural to want alone time but also to be a part of a community.

Being part of a community, the family being the most basic community, builds us emotionally and spiritually, and even physically. For many people, physical progress comes through having an accountability partner, and that is usually found in some type of community. Emotionally, it can be traced all the way back to oxytocin, which is now being called the "love hormone" or "trust hormone." Socially bonding experiences like working together as a community (or even better, playing in the dirt as a community) increase oxytocin and all its benefits.

As I have been able to experience a front yard garden, I have seen firsthand how it can build community. Maybe we don't work together in a garden, but through it, I get the opportunity to meet and most importantly talk and socially bond with people in the community. It isn't just the "hi" and "bye" that most people experience today but an uplifting conversation with someone who many times just lives a couple of houses down from us.

Mother Nature provides so many ways to live a fuller life, not just a healthier life. We have to go to her though. She can't just give us what she wants to give us, which includes among other things the feeling of her beauty, a sense of well-being, and her healing capacity through stress reduction and community building. We must go to her with the mindset of working with, and not against, her. We must perform the action; we must go and do. She is more than willing to give us ten times more than what we put in.

Soil—fresh, clean, pleasant, and medicinal!

My wife and I have a morning custom that we try to never miss: conversing about the day's plans and how we are doing while drinking mate. To me, it is a beautiful way to start the day. Yerba mate is a common drink in a couple of countries in South America. My grandparents on my mother's side, being from Argentina, drank it every day. To me, it is something as normal as eating breakfast.

I still remember the first time I tried mate. Every time I saw my grandparents drinking it, I would bug them to let me try it. They would always say the same thing: "Está muy caliente." (It's too hot.) After bugging them enough, I finally got them to let me try it. They had just finished drinking, the water was lukewarm, and the Yerba mate had lost its flavor. It didn't matter—I was super excited to finally try it. I poured a spoonful of sugar on top of the Yerba mate that was in the gourd (the gourd is the vessel that holds the Yerba mate, which is also called the mate. I know, it's kind of confusing). I then poured the lukewarm water that was left in the teapot on top. I put the bombilla, a metal straw, to my mouth and began to drink. It tasted just like sugar water. I loved it!

What I didn't know at that time was that mate tastes nothing like that. Over the years, it has become something that my wife and I drink a couple of times a day without sugar. We drink it in a way that is called amargo, which in English is translated as "bitter." Mate amargo has become quite popular for all the vitamins and minerals that it contains and is now seen all over the world.

Back in those days, just to get some Yerba mate my grandparents had to get it shipped to them. To them, it was worth the cost, and I completely understand why. Not only does it provide precious vitamins and minerals, but it brings us together as people.

As I was putting our trusty mate (a gourd wrapped in leather with three leather legs to hold it upright) and the Thermos away, I looked over and said, "Hey Verena, Matías, can you help me? I have something I need to do at Ana's house. It is difficult to do alone." The answer didn't come quickly, but slowly, I heard a "sure" from Verena, and a couple of seconds later, Matías also said, "Yes."

Awesome! With the help of my kids, my composting chore was going to be a lot more efficient. The last time I did it alone, I had to hold open a bag (previously used to hold fifty pounds of potatoes) with one hand while my other hand maneuvered a shovel full of "black gold" into the bag, and not all over the ground. Not an easy task when you are working solo.

With their help, I could focus on the shovel and make sure all of the precious "black gold" made it straight into the potato bag.

I have to say, I have a pretty neat composting system. There are four parts to it, the first two parts are two five gallon buckets with holes drilled throughout the sides and their bottoms cut out. The bottoms are tied together with wire, making about a three-foot-long tube with holes all around it. The third part is just a normal plastic milk crate, and the fourth part is the fifty-pound potato bag.

"You all ready?" I asked them as I grabbed the keys to our house and to their grandmother Ana's, who lived about a block away. "It's time to go and play in the dirt." Though my kids were almost tired of hearing that, this was the first time they were helping me with this satisfying work called play. We got to Ana's, said hello to her, and then I went out back to prepare the shovels.

Once I was ready, I called the kids out to help.

"Dad, what are we going to do?" Verena asked. "Today I need your help with the compost."

"Eeeew! That stinky stuff?" Verena asked.

They'd only seen the stuff that goes into the first tube made of two buckets. At our house, we put everything organic in a different container that sits right next to the trash can. We throw in the parts of vegetables we don't eat, eggshells, used charcoal, and even paper receipts (after the totals have been inserted into our homemade budget in Microsoft Excel). When the container gets full, I throw the contents into the first bucket, and since we don't have a lot of dry material, sometimes it will start to stink.

"No, I need your help with the last part only. Then, all the other playing I can do alone," I told Verena while she looked at me with a weird smile. "Playing?" she asked.

As I took a black plastic tarp off of the plastic milk crate, I said, "All I need you two to do is hold open this bag while I dump this black gold into it."

"Black gold? What are you talking about, Dad?"

"I am talking about this beautiful smelling soil here in this plastic crate."

"Wow, it does smell good!" Verena said.

"Yup, this is the almost finished product. What I am going to do now is mix it up one last time and place it in this potato bag that you're holding open in order to let it finish its cycle so we can then mix it into our garden beds."

"Wow! All that multicolored stuff we bring from the house turns into this black fluffy stuff that smells so fresh, clean, and pleasant?"

I replied, "Yup, isn't that crazy?" as I dropped in the first shovel full of compost that would eventually pass its nutrients into the vegetables that we'd be eating in a couple of months.

This beautiful cycle of life is one of the most important details of our health and well-being. Being able to share that with my kids is incredibly rewarding. Since that first time, my kids have helped me on various occasions, making playing in the dirt not just more enjoyable because I am with people that I care about, but also a little easier.

Humans and soil

When I was a kid, for some reason we just seemed to play in the dirt a lot more. I'm not talking about all that fun time planting a garden; I'm talking about literally playing in the dirt.

Some of my fondest memories as a kid are when I was in the dirt, and I imagine many of you are thinking the same thing.

One memory in particular really stands out, and because it almost felt too fantastical to have really happened, I called my older brother to make sure I hadn't made it all up. And true enough, I hadn't.

When I was young, not more than nine years old, I remember some dirt hills in our backyard. Not just any dirt hills, but the type a dump truck would leave after dumping its enormous load.

My older brother explained that our dad had ordered a couple of loads of dirt that would eventually be spread around so the grass he was planning to plant would be on more level ground.

Those hills were a perfect place to play in the dirt. My two older brothers and I decided that we were going to be ants.

The dirt was soft and easy to thrust our shovels into it, and we started what would become a series of tunnels. I began at the bottom of the little dirt mound while one of my older brothers walked to the top and started digging at the center.

"Let's meet in the middle," I called to him.

After the first couple of shovel loads, I had a nice indention in the side of the hill; nothing I could sneak into, but it was about two feet wide and half a foot deep. I kept on thrusting that handy tool of mine into the somewhat soft dirt, taking out loads of dirt. With the dirt not being too hard, I was making great progress. Soon enough, I had dug out a cave where I could fit half of my body. But with each shovel load, it was becoming harder and harder to drag out the dirt and throw it to the side.

I got on my belly and squeezed into the tunnel with my shovel, crawling in military-style. Due to the angle, I thrust the shovel with a lot less strength, and I then had to drag myself out backward, throw the dirt to the side of the hill, and squeeze back in, each time going a little bit farther. And each time, it was just a little bit darker.

Soon, it became too dark to see in front of me. Blindly, I continued working diligently.

Suddenly, there was a light from above. My older brother had broken through from the top. I couldn't wait to enter from the bottom and climb out the top.

All that work—I mean playing—and we'd made our first tunnel connection.

One tunnel became two, then three, and we kept playing and digging and crawling until we had five connected tunnels, all meeting in the middle. We could enter any one of them and come out on a totally different spot on the hill.

We were ants, going in one side and coming out another. We would push our way up out of the middle tunnel that reached the top and slide down. Every time we did this, the low tunnels became just slightly weaker, until one of my older brothers, who was belly crawling through one of the tunnels, felt a sudden heavy weight fall onto his back.

"Get me out of here!" he cried out.

One of the tunnels had collapsed on top of him. We ran over and saw his feet sticking out the front of the tunnel. We grabbed them and pulled him out, and as we did, the other tunnels collapsed. Suddenly our anthill was no more.

Talk about fun! Those were awesome times to be a kid. Most mothers and even some fathers out there reading this might be thinking, "How in the world did their parents let them do that? That is so dangerous!" Maybe, though probably not, and how thankful I am for my parents and their willingness to let us use our imaginations to the fullest. Kids digging, making their own personal ant hill…priceless!

But priceless in more than just memories. What did that accomplish back then, back when I was a little kid getting myself "dirty"? I remember dirt in my mouth, all over my hands, underneath my fingernails, in my little scrapes that I collected from falling off the bike, climbing trees to the tippy top, and playing with other "toys" like shovels, hand saws, hammers, and nails.

What was that all doing for me? Was it just for my enjoyment? Was it just fun and games? No, those fun and games had a huge impact on my health and truly on my life, not just emotionally but in every possible physical way.

My brothers and I were building our physical strength by playing with earth, one of the heaviest substances on the planet. No, we were not complaining about having to shovel dirt and throw it to the side. We had decided to do it and we were having a blast while at the same time building core musculature that was going to help us live pain-free for many years into the future.

By physically being outside with my hands and face and hair and clothes all in the dirt, I was better off. I was not just building a physically strong body from the core (which is the most important) to the extremities, but I was building long-lasting strength on many fronts without even knowing it. Dirt, and all it consists of, builds us. Much of fertile soil's makeup is alive, bacteria being one major component of fertile soil that makes us stronger in so many ways.

Jack Gilbert, author of *Dirt Is Good*, gave a fair warning when he said:

"Most of the bacteria we encounter on a daily basis, and those that reside in and on our bodies, are not just friendly but even essential for keeping us alive. We exterminate them at our peril. In our zeal to vanquish all those classical plagues, we have inadvertently unleashed Pandora's box of modern plagues—the array of slow-killing, miserable, chronic health problems that have become prevalent across the modern world: obesity, asthma, allergies, diabetes, celiac disease, irritable bowel syndrome, multiple sclerosis, rheumatoid arthritis, and many others."

Because of the germ theory, people started to believe the best way to not get sick was to keep everything as clean as possible. Not just clean but sterile. The idea was to eradicate all bacteria in the home and avoid it at all costs outside. So we went from being encouraged to go outside and play, which would almost always involve the dirt, to if we touched the dirt, the first thing that would happen was an adult would pull out some sanitizing solution, which is pretty much alcohol in a gel, and squeeze some on our dirty little hands. Then when we got home, it was straight to the bathroom to wash our hands. Over time, this idea has proved to be somewhat detrimental to our health, and thanks to the hygiene hypothesis, we now know why.

As we enter this world through the birth canal (if it is a natural birth) what we first encounter are the microbes, the bacteria, that live in the mother's birth canal. This is actually a good thing. So, our first interaction with life is with bacteria.

They touch the eyes, mouth, nose, and everywhere else as the baby passes through the birth canal and finally takes its first breath of air with bacteria in it. The baby starts to cry, which is normal and is given to the mother to be calmed. The mother cuddles the baby against her skin, which is also full of bacteria, helping her bundle of joy feel its mother's love, slowly calming the baby down.

Over time, and if we are allowed to, we acquire all sorts of microbes that live on us and in us that actually help us. Some are so important that if we don't have them wandering around our gut or on our skin, we will become sick.

The latest analysis that I found that talks about the number of microbes in our body is pretty interesting:

"[It] puts the ratio at 1.3 microbes per human cell. Thus, an average guy will have about 40 trillion bacterial cells and 30 trillion human cells. Individual differences in body size and gender skew the ratio, but you get the idea: we are a superorganism. You harbor about ten thousand microbial species that altogether weigh about three pounds—the same as your brain."

It goes on to say that:

"…there are at least one hundred microbial genes for every human gene, and they are responsible for many of the biochemical activities associated with your body, ranging from digesting carbohydrates in your food to making some of your vitamins. Importantly, the microbiome is the genome that you can and do change every day. Although our human genome is fixed our whole lives, the genes in our microbiomes change in response to our food, our environment, drugs we take, and even our health." (1)

Before I go on talking about the beauty of playing in the dirt, it is important to understand just a little about our genome.

Our genome is all the genetic material that makes us who we are. Then there is genotype and phenotype. Our genotype is what makes us all unique in our own little way. It doesn't change. Phenotype, on the other hand, does. Our phenotype is the expression or the observable characteristic of our genotype with the

(1) Gilbert, Jack. *Dirt Is Good*. St. Martin's Press.

environment. The first time I read this, it hit me hard. That last part is so important—with the environment. This is where I first understood that my health, my well-being, is completely up to me. I had to take on full responsibility.

My health depends on the environments I put myself into. This includes my internal environment, like the way I talk to myself; my external environment, like what I decide to eat; all the way to where I decide to live. It all comes down to this: If we put ourselves into a healthy environment, both internal and external, we will express health, and we will be healthy. If we put ourselves into an unhealthy environment, we will express the opposite, and we will become sick and unwell. It's simple to understand, yet difficult to put into practice. But it's so worth the effort.

Perfect? Perfect! Let's get back to the importance of putting ourselves into one of the healthiest environments—the dirt.

We have more bacteria in us than we have human cells; as weird as that might sound, it is what we are. At a young age, if allowed, we should have a pretty good balance of bacteria on and in us that work with us.

They take up residence not only in the moist areas of our bodies but also the dry areas helping in the development of our immune system by building a strong defense against all invaders. They have many important jobs, like breaking down fibers and even influencing our mental well-being, as you will read about later on.

Think back to those times. It doesn't matter how old you are when you were a kid and you were complaining to your parents because you didn't want to go outside to either help in the garden or anything else that involved some type of playing in the dirt. Your parents were not only trying to help you learn the importance of a good work ethic but unknowingly, they were building you up from the inside out. They were helping your little body build up a strong self-defense.

Over the years of treating patients, I have noticed two distinct groups of adults. There are those that almost never get sick, and then there are those that every year, almost without exception, will miss appointments because they get sick. Also, almost all of my patients that regularly get sick have some type of allergy, and the ones that don't get sick rarely will have an allergy.

There isn't some crazy reason why I see these very distinct groups of adults. Of course, it isn't just because of one thing they did in their life, but usually, one good thing brings many other good things. For example, playing in the dirt brings nutrient-dense food to the table and the movement of our joints and muscles.

I happen to be one of those people that just doesn't get sick, and now I know why. Before, when people would ask me, "How is it that you never get sick?" I would jokingly answer, "It's because I ate dirt and bugs when I was a kid." Now, I say it not as a joke but in all seriousness because it truly is one of the reasons why I don't get sick when everybody else around me does.

I don't ever remember eating dirt just to eat dirt. I am sure a lot of it made its way into my mouth without me knowing though. Bugs, that is a different story. I do distinctly remember one bug that I ate. As a kid, it was incredible to see how ants would swarm in and out of a hole in the ground; many were leaving, many were entering, and somehow they never smashed right into each other, while at the same time they carried things that were sometimes ten times bigger than they were. I would watch ants work while I played. I don't know why or how that got me to want to see if they were tasty or not, but on various occasions as a kid, I remember taking ants one at a time and chomping them down. I personally remember them to be salty. Gross! Or maybe it is normal? I guess it depends on who you ask.

One of the reasons playing in the dirt is so beneficial is because it exposed us, and exposes our kids today, to all sorts of harmless germs that have complex traits that help train and strengthen our immune system.

When I say immune system, I am not just talking about our defense against foreign enemies; I am also talking about domestic enemies. Remember that we are a host to trillions of microbes, and our defense can become confused if not properly trained just like any army that is outnumbered and surrounded by an enemy soldier that looks very similar to a friendly soldier.

The diverse bacterial world introduced to us through healthy soil trains our immune system to differentiate between friend and enemy, that being domestic or foreign. Without this training, our immune response can confuse a domestic friend as that of an enemy and attack it, causing an inflammatory response in friendly territory. When this happens, it is known as an autoimmune condition, and these conditions range from thyroid issues to diabetes.

It isn't just the wide array of different microbes that train our immune response to identify between self and non-self, or between friend and foe. If we try and keep our world too clean, we can kill off the bacteria, the microbes that guard and protect us. Without the right microbes and what they produce, we have a difficult time controlling inflammation, which will inevitably lead to allergies, asthma, and sensitivities, like gluten intolerance, just to name one.

You might get the idea that inflammation is bad. On the contrary, the activation of the inflammatory response when needed is one of the many important functions of our immune system. A well-trained immune system will use the proper amount of inflammation in the proper place. How do we know how much inflammation is needed? Good question. I can't answer that, but a strong, well-trained immune system can and will. It's one less thing we have to worry about.

One way to make sure that the immune system is able to control inflammation is to first expose it to as many diverse bacteria as possible. Second, deprive the inflammation producing bacteria of their food, which are, seed oils, trans fats and refined sugars. Third, feed the inflammation-fighting bacteria in the gut the proper food. That is why it is so important to eat chemical-free, nutrient-dense fruit, chemical-free, nutrient-dense vegetables and most importantly properly raised meats.

Not only do we have more inflammation-fighting bacteria in our gut when we feed it properly, but when this bacteria takes up residence in our gut we become less susceptible to infection because of the complex communities they form.

It is neat how Jack Gilbert, in his book *Dirt Is Good*, uses seeds and trees as an example when explaining this. As always, nature knows best.

"Think of it like trying to plant seeds in a mature forest rather than on bare soil: it's hard for the new plants to get a foothold under the canopies of the existing trees. The same principle applies to the microbiome, where the complex interrelationships between the anaerobic microbes that develop over time just don't leave a lot of open ecological niches for new microbes coming in to invade."

Gut bacteria and our well-being

A couple of pages back, I mentioned that bacteria in the gut can even influence our well-being. How in the world can those little critters influence our well-being? Great question!

Most, using their logic, would think that our central nervous system controls our well-being, that it all starts in the brain where our thoughts form. In many ways, they are correct. However, it is a lot more than just thought formation. Everything that comes before and after the formation of the thought is very important in our well-being. The nerve impulses and the chemicals, including all those hormones that we hear so much about today, doing their best job adapting to the environment we put them in, have a lot to do with our mood.

All those chemicals that our brain tells our body to build are not our special little chemicals. Those same chemicals that we build are also built and consumed by the bacteria in our gut. For example, Candida, which is found in a healthy gut microbiome builds 5-hydroxytryptophan which is a precursor to serotonin. Serotonin is known as one of the happy hormones. It is believed to help with mood, sleep, and memory among other things. Other bacteria build dopamine, the other feel-good hormone, while others build noradrenaline and others, acetylcholine. All very important neurotransmitters.

When we can't build enough serotonin—for example, when we are chronically stressed—our gut bacteria can lend us a hand. Serotonin built in the gut, which is mainly used for helping regulate intestinal movement, can pass the blood-brain barrier and give us a hand, lift us up, and influence our well-being.

Our gut also has its own nervous system, the enteric nervous system, sometimes called "the second brain" because it has been shown to be able to function without the central nervous system. The central nervous system and enteric nervous system are constantly in communication through the vagus nerve.

Another neurotransmitter built by the bacteria in the gut is GABA. GABA is a very important inhibitory neurotransmitter that also plays a role in our mood and well-being. The communication coming and going through the vagus nerve keeps both systems on top of each other. If one is not on its game, the other will know. If the proper amount of GABA is not being built, that being too much or too little by the bacteria in the gut, the central nervous system will feel those effects through the vagus nerve, therefore affecting how our brain is building and using GABA, which will affect our overall mood. If our gut is not on its game, it makes it hard for the brain to be on its best game.

All the way back when I was a kid outside playing in the dirt, I had no idea what was forming inside of me. I had no idea of the army of white blood cells and bacteria building up my defenses against all enemies foreign and domestic. I had no idea that there were bacteria taking up residence in my gut, building important neurotransmitters that would allow me to develop. These things just happened naturally because I was allowed to get dirty.

It's not too late if you haven't made it a priority to get into contact with soil. Now is the time! Dig your hands in the dirt and don't wash them afterward; instead, make yourself a peanut butter and jelly sandwich and eat it with your hands, no need for a fork.

For those of you with kids, what can you do? I go back to a great question that was asked in the book *Dirt Is Good*:

"Should I take my kids to a farm? Yes, as early in their life as possible, and as frequently as possible. And while there, let them stroke as many animals as they want and even rub their faces up against the ones that will let them. Let them enjoy all the dirt, mud, grit, and dust they can find. Rolling in hay won't hurt. Feeding critters by hand is fun. The only word of caution is that you might want to stop them from eating any poop they find on the floor."

If you can't make it to a farm, Jack Gilbert gives another great recommendation.

"Let your kid play in (and even eat) dirt. Soil is microbial heaven, with more than a billion bacterial cells per gram, and many fungi and viruses as well. Unless there's lots of animal poop around the soil (which would be a bit gross), you can relax in knowing the soil contains very few organisms that could make your child sick. It is a great source and a great opportunity to expose children to a complex microbial community that will help train their immune system."

This might sound difficult. It can be a total paradigm shift. Maybe your whole life you were told clean, clean, clean. Don't, you will get dirty! Put your shoes on before you go outside! Wash your hands! Or if you have kids, maybe your kids just don't want to go outside because the iPad or screen is too enticing.

I completely understand if your kids don't care to play in the dirt. This is not easy to write because I am not the best example. I would love it to be different, but I don't have that many opportunities to get my kids out in the dirt. And the few opportunities that I do have, my kids make it known that they have little desire to go outside and play in the dirt. How am I going to write about something that I struggle to do personally?

Well, even though I truly want them to be outside in the dirt with me so they can build strong immune systems among many other benefits, it just isn't how it is at this moment. But that's not enough of a reason to not write about this now. It is too important that even though I am not walking the walk as I would like to, these things need to be shared.

"Our bodies evolved in a world teeming with microbes. They are in us, on us, all around us—without them, we could not survive…That's why these trips to a farm, or even—if possible— engaging in local farming projects or gardening can be so vital." (2)

Let's get out there and play in the dirt with our kids!

(2) Gilbert, Jack. *Dirt Is Good*. St. Martin's Press.

The garden and meditation

It sucked, it hurt, and it tore me apart to finally become aware of my situation and begin to understand that I was having trouble coping with my day-to-day life due to my toxic emotional state.

I knew it deep inside but I just didn't want to believe it. So much fighting within my own mind. However, I continued to think, to believe that things would somehow get better. There was one moment early on, about thirteen years ago when I was in my mid-twenties when I first started to experience this toxic emotional state that it got to the point where I broke my hand out of frustration.

I did not understand what was wrong, what was the problem. What was causing me to think such negative, detrimental thoughts? Not knowing where to throw the frustration, I started to punch the floor, hoping that the padding and carpet were enough of a cushion. Not even close. I broke my hand trying to get rid of the frustration! I know exactly what bone it was now: the fifth metacarpal at its distal end. It was so painful that I was not able to catch a pass while playing basketball for a couple of weeks. Of course, I lied to my dad when he asked me why I was trying to catch the ball with one hand. I don't remember what I told him, but I know it wasn't the truth.

This toxic emotional state was sucking the life, the energy, and everything else you can think of right out of me. It was a bottomless pit of quicksand that was constantly pulling me in, and it felt as if there was no one there to help me out. For years, I slowly allowed myself to create an internal environment that was not in harmony with who I truly was.

How did this happen? How did I let it get to this point? My internal dialogue had become completely toxic, and it was literally killing me. I would talk to myself in ways that I would never talk to another person.

I was living with an almost insurmountable amount of self-made stress. I would ask myself:

"Why doesn't the heart attack come so I can just leave? I am stressed to the max. Come on heart attack, do your wonders."

People who know me, know that my hands shake a little. It got to the point of it becoming difficult to type on the computer. I shake now as I write this because this stuff is just plain hard to write about.

How is it possible? Such destructive internal dialogue had destroyed absolutely any desire to live.

For those that this resonates with, I hope this helps you realize that you are not alone in any way, shape, or form. You are not alone when you go through the times that seem endless and horrible and worthless. We all go through them to some degree, even if it doesn't look like it on the outside.

Some might say, "Man, that's nothing!"

Some might say, "Man, how did you get through it?"

In the zone

Well, there is hope. It started in 2009 when I returned to my roots. Literally and figuratively. I was reading a lot of material about modern survivalism. This was during my last year at Palmer College of Chiropractic in Davenport, Iowa. I tell you the place because it does have something to do with it. While studying modern survivalism, and how to prepare for what life can throw at you, the garden kept coming up. The garden was and still is, a great way to prepare for those unexpected events that we don't want to happen, but inevitably will.

At that point in my evolution in modern survivalism, I was preparing a "bug out bag," which is a seventy-two-hour kit in a backpack that is always ready to go. I had built four shelves in the basement out of wood that a fellow student had given me and was using a bookshelf that had another four shelves that had come with the house. They were full of cans of fruit and vegetables and prepared soups. I had water stored. I even had some 9mm ammo stored.

We were using the method of buying one more can each time we went to the supermarket, and it was filling up fast. I would buy a box of fifty rounds of 9mm ammo when the boxes were available because at the time, it was pretty difficult to find them. It made me feel good that we had a little extra food for emergencies and that I had a way to defend my family.

We also asked the bakeries in the supermarkets if they would give us the used and empty three and five-gallon buckets of cake topping that were left over. We got hold of six of them. I cleaned them out as thoroughly as possible and we started to fill them up with black beans, lentils, macaroni, oatmeal, dried potato flakes, and powdered milk by buying an extra bag of one item each time we went to the supermarket.

It started to feel like we could take on a mini-disaster. I also had bought a couple of silver coins to keep inflation at bay. I say a couple because as a student, money was a very rare thing.

But something was missing. It was the garden. I needed to return to my roots. We didn't have any place to plant, and the place we were living in was a rental. Well, that didn't stop me.

As we would go on walks, I would find wood planks thrown out in the trash. I would ask the owners if I could take them, and they would always say, yes. After a couple of weeks, I had enough wood to make myself a nice planter box that was about three feet long by one foot wide and about one foot deep. It also had two legs. The backside sat on the windowsill, and the front was supported by the two legs. I also found two big flower pots that had been thrown out by our neighbors. I had a pretty big planter box and two big flower pots for my very first garden. I was stoked!

I bought some flower potting mix, tomato seeds, and red bell pepper seeds. I planted the seeds in eggshells, cracked in half, and filled up the planter box and two flower pots with the store-bought potting mix. Those that know Iowa understand it is perfect for growing anything, and that was a good thing for me.

I was so excited that I planted way too many seeds. A couple of days later, I saw little plants poking out of the dirt in the eggshells. There were too many plants for the little space that I had, but I was too happy to worry about that. It felt great preparing, working, and finally seeing the plants grow.

Preparing, working, and just watching those little plants brought me to the present moment. I was in the now when I was doing those things. I wasn't worried about my past, I wasn't anxious about my future, and I definitely did not focus on all the negative comments I said to myself almost nonstop. It felt incredible to have nothing else on my mind. I was physically active, but my mind was still.

At that time in my life, I wasn't just worried about the past, the anxiety of the future, and the negative comments I so often told myself. I was also in classes as a full-time job and was studying pretty much every other minute I had to prepare for tests. It was brutal, and I didn't allow any time to just be in the now. I lost a lot of precious time with my family, not because I was never with them physically but because of the little time I was with them, I was mentally in the future. I was worrying about the next test. It was a very difficult time.

I had to study a lot to get through Palmer College. There were months when my daily schedule would begin between midnight and 1 a.m. so I could study until about 6 a.m. I would then get ready for school and make my lunch. I would ride my bike to school to start classes at around 7 a.m., and each time I had a break between classes, I would go to the library and find a cubicle so I could continue to study until classes were over. Between 6 p.m. and 7 p.m., I would ride home, eat with my family, chill for a little while with the family, and by 8 p.m. be in bed to wake up again at midnight.

Those difficult times of being a graduate student, combined with the negative self-talk, were a ticking time bomb. I found that the garden was what turned off the timer on that bomb. It brought me back to reality, to the now. It was meditation at its best.

I didn't find the meditative qualities of gardening until the start of my third year at Palmer College. When I began that little planter box garden in Iowa, for the first time in a long time, and of course only in short bursts of time, I would leave the past behind. I would put the future in context, and my mind of constant chatter would stop. I would just be present! Wow, what a gift it was! What I started to notice was that those short bursts of time would linger on, and I was more present after working in the garden, after playing in the dirt. And when I stopped working in the garden, I wouldn't revert to my old self. It changed how I interacted with people, as well as with myself.

The short moments where I would come home and take fifteen minutes to water and enjoy the plants was a lifesaver. It put me in the zone; it was meditation, the altered state of consciousness that we all need to find to bring us back to the now.

We have many moments of being in the zone in everyday life. A simple example is what I am seeing right now. I am in my brother's dining room, and there is a big window in the kitchen that lets you enjoy their backyard. I see peace. My brother is outside with his little daughter. He is pushing her in a swing, and it looks so beautiful. It feels like he is enjoying the now, those moments that we all need to experience on a daily basis. Our health depends on it. We must set aside time every day to allow ourselves to be in the zone. The word commonly used for this is meditation. But meditation does not have to be you sitting cross-legged on a pillow on the ground, controlling your breathing. Mediation can be found in many ways, like my brother completely in the now, focused on swinging his daughter outside on a beautiful humid day.

Meditation, being in the zone, having that altered state of consciousness, is all about being in the moment. If you play sports, you know what being in the zone is. It is that moment where everything just goes right. I have felt it two times in my life playing basketball.

It is a majestic experience. I must have been sixteen when I first experienced it. I was on a church basketball team. We played against other churches. You might think, well, that doesn't sound too competitive. However, it became quite competitive, and we even had crowds that came and watched the games. They were great experiences.

There was one game where we played a church that had brought the majority of the local high school talent onto their team. They were the best team, and we were playing them in the finals. I have always been more of a defensive player in basketball. My favorite part of the game is rebounds, offensive rebounds being my main focus. In this game, I found myself in the zone. I can't tell you what I did to get into the zone, but I could not do anything wrong defensively. The game was intense and finished off with a bang. Their biggest player, a guy bigger and better than I, had the ball, and he was determined to dunk it. I vividly remember that he got a running start, jumping off one foot toward the rim, and me jumping off my two feet, straight up. He had the momentum, however, when we struck each other in the air, I did not move. I stayed my ground in the air, blocking the dunk, and the other bigger and stronger player fell to the ground. I could not believe it at that moment, and it is difficult to believe now, but it happened. I was in the zone. I was in an altered state of consciousness where anything was possible.

On another occasion, and on a totally different team, I remember playing against another team that was clearly better than the one I was on.

They knew it, too. They let us know by trash-talking and playing as if they didn't care at the beginning. Well, for some reason that put me in the zone. As I stated above, I am usually not an offensive player, but the team I was playing on didn't have any offense. Somehow, I was able to dribble, drive, and score with ease against bigger and better players. Everything I shot would go in. An experience that has never been duplicated. Again, it is still hard to believe that I was able to drive and score effortlessly, but it happened, and we won that game because I was in the zone. I was in an altered state of consciousness, totally focused on the moment, totally in the present.

I tell you this to help you imagine what playing in the dirt can do for you, what gardening can do for you. It is one of the best ways to meditate, to put yourself in the zone, to have that altered state of consciousness, to be in the present, the now.

Finding the time in this modern world

For some odd reason we are making our lives busier and busier, making it harder and harder to find time to be in the present. I first experienced that crazy busyness during those grueling times at Palmer College. There was no time for anything it seemed, and that made the internal dialogue that much more negative. I couldn't find a way out.

I eventually graduated with honors with the help of my wonderful wife and those fifteen minutes at a time that I had to enjoy my super tiny garden. However, I wasn't even able to enjoy graduation because of my constant worrying about the future and negative internal dialogue.

In my last trimester, I was able to work in the clinic of a chiropractic physician and learn as much as I could from him. It was a great experience where I followed him around while he treated patients. To be able to do this, I had to pack everything up and move my family back out west. When I finished my final trimester, I learned that I had to be at the graduation ceremony to get my diploma; they couldn't just send it to me in the mail. The cost of flying back to Davenport, Iowa with the family would be steep.

But I hadn't put all that hard work in for those three-and-a-half years for nothing. I forked up the cash that I didn't have and bought round-trip tickets for the whole family. Luckily, our good friends let us stay in their home for the few days we were there.

The graduation was all kind of a blur. Between my negative internal environment and the stress of finishing school with a huge amount of debt on my shoulders with really no clear way of paying it off, put me in a state where I was just not me. Well, I hadn't been me for a while, to tell you the truth.

I tried to fake it as much as I could by trying to enjoy the graduation, however, when it was all over, it hit me like a brick wall. Nothing had changed. I didn't feel any different even though I had just received my diploma and I was officially a doctor in chiropractic. I was hoping to feel something, some type of relief, some type of hope. But nope, nothing. It hit me hard and knocked me down, and I wasn't able to get up.

After graduation, we didn't have anything special planned. My wife wanted to celebrate, and we had every right to. We had just gone through a very arduous journey and made it through to the other side. With my negative internal environment and anxious worry for the future, I just couldn't get myself to enjoy the moment.

Instead, the opposite happened; I ruined the situation for everybody. I couldn't find the way to explain to my wife what I was going through, my feeling of inadequacy, self-doubt, and anxiety for a future burdened with the pressure of a huge load of debt. This frustrated her, and to top it off, I wouldn't spend any money to celebrate because we didn't have any money to celebrate with. So, we ended up eating Burger King in the car. I cried of sadness and frustration that night instead of joy, as I should have. I can almost feel it as I write this. A very difficult moment, which should have been a beautiful one in our lives together.

With school over and the state jurisprudence test passed, I was officially working as a chiropractic physician in the state of Nevada—with the same negative internal dialogue and anxiety as before.

A lifestyle – gardening and meditation

One thing I have always loved is reading and learning, even in those dark times in my life. With school over, I had the chance to really dive into things that I truly enjoyed. I got my hands on whatever I could that involved permaculture and wellness-based living.

Through those very difficult times, the garden is what brought me back to the present, putting me into that altered state of consciousness.

Before I continue, I have to say that I still have hard times today. Not everything is like a bed of roses. I am constantly trying to learn and improve who I am. I still have hard times, and though they don't reach so low of a point, they are there.

In Las Vegas, I got a great opportunity. The climate wasn't as garden-friendly as Iowa, but I was up to the task. In Iowa, I had my two flower pots and small wooden box made out of scrap wood. In Las Vegas, I now had a quarter-acre of desert to work on. It was about as dead as dead can be. That did not stop me though. I got my hands on anything related to desert permaculture, from ways to harvest and use the little rain that did fall, to the local trees and plants that I could use to speed up the process of converting my quarter-acre of desert into a paradise. That is what I told myself at least.

First things first. I took my trusty Makita cordless power drill that I had from all those years of working construction and made a three-tier composting system out of old scrap plywood that I found around the yard. I then grabbed a pickax and a shovel and started picking out earthworks that would help me take advantage of the little rain that did fall in the region.

Doing those tasks, I was in complete meditation. I was fully in the moment. I felt present. I can't say I felt joy or something special, but I felt present. I didn't feel anxious or speak to myself in a sick manner. I picked and shoveled out dirt that was sometimes so hard that it took me hours to just dig a couple of inches down. If you have ever worked with caliche, you know what I am talking about. It is like trying to go through rock. This was in the middle of the summer, where the Las Vegas heat can easily reach 115 degrees Fahrenheit.

I remember going into work on a Monday and the other chiropractic physician I worked with asked me how I got through the weekend. The Saturday before had been the hottest day of the year. I remember he told me that it had reached 117 degrees. I hadn't realized it but I had worked outside pretty much all day Saturday with the sun beating on me. I was able to achieve such a beautiful altered state of focus, of consciousness, that the heat didn't even bother me.

In arid regions, there is a lot of digging because you have to plant everything in sunken beds to take advantage of the small amount of rainfall. I dug all my keyhole sunken garden beds and my swales on contour, with a pick and shovel. I also got in contact with a local tree trimming company and they started to bring truckloads of chipped wood in. Free mulch is another important aspect of desert gardening. I planted a windbreak of local corkscrew mesquite trees with a couple of inches of mulch around them. I was also able to get my hands on a mandarin tree, an orange tree that I had planted from a seed of an orange that I had bought in Walmart while living in Iowa. It also made the trip out west with us. That tree is now planted in my aunt's backyard. I also had a plum tree and apricot tree, a peach tree that my grandma had planted from seed, and a pomegranate tree. These were all planted on the downside of the swales I had picked and shoveled out. I planted vegetables in the sunken beds, laying inches of mulch in between each little plant.

My dad and I constructed a dome out of wood that we used as a chicken coop where we had chickens and a rooster. A beautiful system was slowly coming alive.

The quarter-acre desert was truly turning into a desert paradise in my eyes. Local resilient trees were placed to help the system grow and develop with other fruit trees on the lower sides of the swales, taking advantage of the small amount of rain we got. My sunken beds had some fertile soil that was brought in from an outside source, while I waited for the compost I was making from house scraps, dry leaves, and grass clippings from my dad's house to finish evolving.

Over time, I started to see some results of my playing in the dirt as small amounts of fruit from the trees started to blossom, the garden beds began to produce a few vegetables, and the chickens started to lay eggs. A very small portion of our diet was coming from our backyard. It wasn't just the physical results either. Even though I was still plagued with anxiety and had negative internal dialogue, I found the internal peace necessary to continue because of that little quarter acre.

I write about it now and it seems so nice, but those were very hard times for me internally. I would get home from work and say hi to my wife and kids and almost immediately go outside to work in the garden. Sometimes, the work was just me looking around, allowing myself to enjoy the present of what I was building. Those few minutes of garden meditation were crucial in those moments in my life; back then I didn't understand how important they truly were. That quarter-acre paradise lasted about three years.

We ended up moving for various reasons. Yup, I know…all that playing in the dirt and now moving on. It was time. We found a place, but it had pretty much no yard. We had just a little area where we could plant.

That didn't stop me. I loaded all the compost I had made over the years at the quarter-acre lot into the back of my pickup and took it to the new place, where I was going to continue to plant what I could. At the new place, I didn't have the space like before, but I took advantage of what I did have. While there, I got some of the best harvests of cherry tomatoes and Armenian cucumbers ever. The best tasting cantaloupe I ever ate was also grown in that little space.

The garden has continued to help me with the day-to-day challenges my mind likes to play on me. My garden now is made up of five planter boxes in a backyard that is pure cement and an area that is between the street and sidewalk in front of my house that is about eight feet by eight feet in the city of Rosario, Argentina.

Rosario is known for its fertile land, but the little space I have was used as a parking spot for a vehicle and was full of broken brick and rock. With the help of a trusty shovel, I continue to find those times where I can be here-and-now. I look for those moments that have helped me so much and continue to help me. Those are the moments where I can play in the dirt, helping

Mother Nature bring back—if just a small piece of land—the soil life that is needed to heal and provide my family with some nutrient-dense food we can eat to help us stay strong and healthy.

The altered state of consciousness that the garden helped me achieve would continue into the kitchen on many occasions. While in Las Vegas, it happened quite often. One way was with the Armenian cucumbers. Because we had so many of them, I had to think of ways to consume as many as possible. We also gave a lot of them to family and friends.

Those moments that helped me so much started with me enjoying the view the plants gave me, then with a knife, cutting two cucumbers off the vine, then slicing them small enough for my kids to enjoy, and adding just a little flavor with Himalayan salt and freshly-squeezed lemon juice. Not only did I love it, my kids ate it up like candy. What more could a father ask for than seeing his kids enjoying nutrient-dense food from the garden? And that feeling of being here-and-now continued while I slowly sliced the cucumbers, seasoned them, and finally offered them to my kids. Those are beautiful memories.

It also happened with kale. We had so much that we didn't know what to do. It was a good problem to have. Again, I would start by just being outside and cutting the biggest leaves one at a time and placing them in a bowl. Once I had enough, I would go into the kitchen and wash each leaf, placing them into the blender where I also had cut some type of fruit. No, I didn't just grab the whole bunch and run it under the flow of water from the faucet in the kitchen. I took each individual leaf and washed it. Sounds tedious, but how relaxing it was to take that time, and how it prolonged the feeling of being in the now. I continue to do it today with beet leaves and Swiss chard from the garden, or when I buy beet leaves, Swiss chard, and lettuce from the local market here in Argentina. I am a lot better now, and much of it has to do with the garden.

People are living a lifestyle that is just too busy for anything. One of the common complaints or excuses is "I don't have enough time." I had, and still have, pretty much the same rigorous schedule as most people, but I find time for these activities to be outside playing in the dirt and then bringing that play into the kitchen, where I continue to experience the positive effects of the garden while I prepare and cook for my family and friends.

Let's talk about something different for a second. One of my favorite things to experience is watching family and friends enjoy something that I cooked, and that's made even more joyful when I'm able to use ingredients that come straight from the garden, or a source that I trust. Playing in the garden, then preparing and cooking, and finally enjoying it with friends and family has got to be one of the most healthful activities that is being lost in modern societies. It seems that there just isn't enough time for it. Or is it that we don't have our priorities set right? It's a question we should all ask ourselves.

From my first personal garden of two flower pots and a homemade planter box in 2009, I have had beautiful opportunities to plant gardens in different states and even different countries, and each time it has helped me focus on one task at a time, helping me leave the past behind, put the future in context, and force my internal dialogue to close its mouth. I treasure those moments and know they have helped me internally more than I will ever comprehend. I look forward to the opportunities that I will have in the future to play in the dirt and to continue to give my mind a break. I have come a long way, and I still have a long way to go. I still struggle with my internal dialogue. I still worry about my financial future, but I am in a lot more control now.

As I have continued to grow and learn about the importance of being in the present moment, I have come across different methods of meditation that I now include in my own lifestyle. Also, I now take time almost every day to sit and focus on my breath and affirm certain beliefs. I sit and try to be still in mind, body, and spirit. Doing this has also made my gardening experience even more enjoyable and even more therapeutic.

One of the different methods of meditation that I have learned about is mindfulness and the importance of gratitude in the meditation practice. This is something that I have included more and more while I garden.

Mindfulness in the garden

Our brain is indescribably incredible, but its main mission is to keep us alive. It will do anything to help us see another day, even be willing to do us harm in the long run if it keeps us alive today.

This is a good thing, first because we get to live another day, and second because usually what stresses our ecosystem comes in short-term events. These are events that last minutes to maybe days, but usually minutes. Those short bursts, when our brain has to keep us alive, end up not causing us harm because they are very short-lived, and we have systems in place that neutralize the damage and are able to rebuild and recuperate quickly. The problem is when the events are not short-lived.

When we live a lifestyle that provides the proper internal and external environments to our ecosystem of cells, we become miraculously blessed with incredible health that most in the modern world have never experienced. I didn't say that there aren't people out there that don't feel great. What I am saying is that they could feel even better. I say this because the modern world is just plain overflowing with too many physical, emotional, chemical, noise, light, and other types of stressors out there.

We were supposed to live a natural, healthy lifestyle until the next short-lived danger arrives. That was how it worked not too long ago. We'd supply our bodies with the proper internal and external environments, and when danger arrived in that short burst, we hopefully survived and returned to live a natural, healthy lifestyle.

Today, with our self-made, overly stressful lives, we put ourselves in constant "danger," and our brains are constantly on the alert. I put danger in quotation marks because the majority of the danger is self-inflicted, like eating products from the center aisles in supermarkets, constantly worrying about economic situations, exaggerating and not letting it go when someone cuts you off while driving to work, and letting those events run over and over again in our minds, making you anxious and even angry the whole day.

We live in a world that is overly stressed, constantly looking for the next thing that supposedly will give us a life of a little more luxury instead of just living well with what nature provides. With this constant stressful battle, our brain forms neural pathways. As we use these neural pathways, they become more sensitized. The brain likes this because it makes its job easier, and it doesn't have to work so hard to make decisions. It just uses the most used neural pathways, and with each use it becomes more sensitized, making it more easily used. Over time, it becomes very difficult to change.

This system works great when we are not chronically stressed. When we are stressed, we are not able to make proper conscious decisions, and we begin to form neural pathways that are not what our bodies need to thrive, but what they need to survive, which will eventually result in disease. This is the stress response. Sounds depressing, and well, the way the world is today, it kind of is. It's no wonder that in developed countries, there is more and more depression and anxiety than ever in the history of the world. It shocked me when I read in Mark Manson's *Everything is F*cked: A Book about Hope*.

"Perhaps it can be summed up in one startling fact: the wealthier and safer the place you live, the more likely you are to commit suicide."

Those negative neural pathways can become so sensitized that it can get to a point where it is pretty much all the brain knows. It becomes hard to be grateful for anything or just to see the good in things. When you view the glass as half-empty all the time, you can't expect to immediately start seeing it as half-full.

However, just as the brain can form neural pathways that take us down a destructive path, it can also do the opposite and form neural pathways that take us down a path of health and well-being if we regularly put it in the adequate internal and external environments.

The proper internal environment is an environment of gratitude. It is not so easy to build when we are in a stressed environment. How can we put ourselves in a situation where it is easy to be grateful? The garden, of course!

In the garden, there are just so many things to be grateful for: the seeds, plants, fruit, sun, rain, trees, and the soft, pleasant, and cool soil. It is a very special place to be grateful for life as we see the cycle of life in the plants we nurture. Just as a plant's life is a miracle, ours is also. In the garden, or really in nature, by just looking around, there are many things to be grateful for.

As we put ourselves in the zone, that altered state of consciousness while we garden, it becomes even easier to be grateful. As we focus on a seed, for example, it becomes much easier to be thankful for that seed, and as we take the time to be thankful for that one seed, it helps us enter the zone.

In the garden, we also get to be mindful and grateful using all five senses. It's not just being grateful for the soil, but while digging through it with our bare hands, we can feel it and be mindful of it. We can mindfully breathe in the fresh air and smell the lovely flowers, plants, and soil. We can listen mindfully to the birds and the rustling of leaves in the wind around us. We can mindfully enjoy the explosion of flavor in our mouth from a fruit harvested with our own hands. We can mindfully experience and participate in the creation of life and death through a plant, being that more grateful for our short life we have to enjoy on earth.

The garden is a perfect place to let everything go and immerse yourself in a healthy environment. It's an environment where one can slowly but surely change the neuronal pathways from stress and destruction to peace and creation. Using the garden to help see all that there is to be grateful for will help cultivate positive neuronal pathways.

James Allen phrased it beautifully when he said:

"A man's mind may be likened to a garden, which may be intelligently cultivated or allowed to run wild; but whether cultivated or neglected, it must, and will, bring forth. If no useful seeds are put into it, then an abundance of useless weed seeds will fall therein, and will continue to produce their kind."

As I continue to play in the dirt, I am not only playing but I mindfully play. I consciously try to cultivate seeds that will bring forth good fruit and not just let any seed cultivate in my mind, producing weeds. I am definitely not perfect, and I still have hard days, but they are much milder and bearable with my mindful playing in the garden. I not only wake up and start my day with gratitude for another day, but the garden re-enforces that gratitude as I touch the soil, plant seeds, smell the fresh air, and water the plants.

I am so grateful for the small planter box garden I have where I can dig my hands into homemade compost. It's where I consciously plant each seed and wait for a bright future of harvestable fruit, and at the same time, not worry if it doesn't happen. I am so grateful for potable water that allows me to water my plants when there isn't enough rain and for the rain when it falls. I am grateful for the ability to save seed and for the sun that gives life to the plants that I nurture. And I am incredibly grateful for the opportunity I have to share this information with you, the reader.

I am grateful for people that came before me and left their words written for me to read and help me understand better what is truly important. For example, the words of Lucius Annaeus Seneca, a Stoic philosopher:

"The founder of the universe, who assigned to us the laws of life, provided that we should live well, but not in luxury. Everything needed for our well-being is right before us, whereas what luxury requires is gathered by many miseries and anxieties. Let us use this gift of nature and count it among the greatest things." - Moral Letters, 119.15b

I've hit low points where I thought there was no way out. I didn't even feel I needed a way out. I got to the point of constant toxic internal dialogue. That first little garden in Bettendorf, Iowa allowed me to focus on one thing: to enter the zone, to meditate, to be here now and enjoy it. It gave me the hope I needed to see a way out and the desire to move in that direction. I am still on that path, and though I sometimes weave a little from the path, I am so grateful for the beautiful opportunity to be able to play in the dirt.

Let's never forget as Ritu Ghatourey said,

"Our mind is a garden, our thoughts are the seeds, we can grow flowers, or we can grow weeds."

Earth and our natural electrical state!

My escape

This was not the first time, and it seemed to always happen for the same reason. This one thing: Anger. It's like I just can't overcome it. I have come so far, and am overcoming so many weaknesses, but this one gets hold of my emotions and won't let go. So, again I allow my emotions to completely take over. I was mad. I was so tired of it all!

I had lost it before, and I did not want to fall into that trap. The anger trap has to be the most vicious cycle you can put yourself into. But I was so disappointed, so mad, so worked up. Why did it happen and why could I not control my emotions? I had to vent, and it had to be now. What could I do?

For me, one of the best ways to vent has been through physical movement to the point of exhaustion. I need to beat myself down physically. I have to suffer. That has been one of my best and most effective ways to overcome anger, the feeling of being deceived, of feeling like a nobody, of feeling like a complete failure.

I had to get out there and crush myself physically. Maybe by crushing myself physically, I can also crush my ego that allows me to get angry and defensive, and all those other negative emotions that 99 percent of the time make the situation worse.

It is past 9 p.m. on a hot humid summer day, but that doesn't matter. In the kitchen, I fill up my water bladder with two liters of filtered water, put on my headphones, plug them into my phone, open up Spotify, and tap on my favorite workout music, good old Dropkick Murphys. I turn up the volume to "too loud," throw my phone in my backpack, and sling it around my shoulders. I don't care about my poor eardrums; I have to block out any negative emotions. I leave the house and all the negative emotions behind.

I stretch my legs and then start out at a nice trot, not crazy fast but moving faster than most people when starting to run. I pick it up at the end of the block and continue at that pace for the next five blocks.

I arrive at a building where some long poles that are normally used as soccer goal posts are stored. I have a key to the building, and I use the poles as weights. Here, I continue to push myself to the point of not being able to lift my arms. My legs twitch and I'm huffing, trying to get enough oxygen to the muscles that are burning.

I love that feeling. It makes me feel alive. The poles are heavy as I do sets of power cleans with burpees in between. I work out until my muscles can't go anymore. Why not? I have to vent.

Once I'm done, just putting the poles back into their places is a job of its own.

My legs and arms are beat, but I feel great. I now head off for a run with intermittent sprints. It feels almost like I am floating, my legs and arms are so light. I sprint a block, then jog a block, and I do this until I reach the beautiful landscape of the Paraná River. When I finish the sprint, it feels like my lungs are on fire, but I am just getting started. Now, at the river there are markers with a perfect distance between them to do intermittent sprinting and running. I continue until I get to the fence where no one enters without paying. I turn around and run back doing the same thing. I am tired but I push, and I love that push. I don't think I have any more to give, but I continue to push myself physically to sprint. I feel that terrible burn in my lungs as I slow down to a fast jog. I finish running next to the Paraná River, through the sand on the beach. It brings me back to the river run I did in San Diego, running in cadence while in Marine Corps boot camp. Great times! Push, don't stop. I make it back to the street and continue to sprint one block and then run a block.

I do this all the way home. I reach home exhausted. But no, I don't go inside. I fall on the grass in front of my house. I take my shoes and socks off and plant my bare feet in the lush green grass and clovers around me. I am not done yet. I finish with three sets of twenty push-ups with twenty seconds of rest in between, all the while jamming to Dropkick Murphys with my shoes and socks off.

Drinking water, sitting on the grass with my toes playing with the long blades of grass, is when it truly sinks in. My feet and hands are in contact with Mother Nature. No rubber sole in between my feet and Mother Nature. I am back to reality. I am physically tired to the max, but I am back; those negative emotions of hate, of anger, of self-worthlessness are gone, and that beautiful cool refreshing feeling of grass between my toes and fingers brings me back to life, the right life. It's the life of not blaming everybody else, of accepting each moment in life with humility.

For so many years I thought it was just the physical exertion that brought me back to the type of life where I can take responsibility for the things I can change— and then change them. In other words, bring me back into focus. However, I have learned over time, that it is not just the exertion but the cool down, and how and where I cool down.

Nature is what grounds me. Earth is what brings me truly back to who I am.

Nature wants to help!

It is incredible how it all works! As you now know, we are part of nature. We're an integral part of the ecosystem and nature wants to help us if we will just let it. And we need her help; we can't make it without her. We will become sick if nature is not an integral part of our life.

We have blocked her out with concrete jungles called cities and plastic barriers called shoes. My feet touching the grass was what my body was truly asking for. Yes, it is good to physically exert ourselves; movement is vital to our health and we should look for opportunities to move as much as possible. At the same time, the earth below us wants to help; it wants to ground us. We just need to prioritize time to accept the invitation.

Another great and beautiful detail of my youth is that I had absolutely no problem accepting the invitation. I constantly played in the dirt and if I wasn't playing in the dirt, I was working in the dirt (also known as playing!) or sitting on the ground watching a tractor play in the dirt.

I remember one specific day as if it was yesterday. It was afternoon in a small town in southern Utah called Parowan. It was one of those days where the sky was completely blue and the temperature was perfect for a pair of jeans and a T-shirt. There was a big lilac bush to the left of the detached garage of my parents' house, which separated our house from the neighbor's. I remember sitting on the grass, not knowing at the time, of course, that I was receiving the life-giving energy of the earth. I was facing my neighbor's house, watching a backhoe tractor tear out concrete steps. It was a lot of concrete, and it was hours of enjoyment for me. I imagine the backhoe operator felt bad, thinking something like,

"What is wrong with that kid? How can he sit there for so long just watching me work?"

I had been there for hours, but to me, it felt like minutes of pure joy. Suddenly, I heard the motor of the tractor lower its RPMs, and through the cab I saw the operator wave me over. I was beyond excited.

"Would you like to sit in the cab while I finish tearing out these steps?" he asked.

Overjoyed, I jumped into the cab and was able to experience firsthand the power of a backhoe tractor. It was an experience I will never forget! I still remember the name of the backhoe operator. It was a beautiful time to be a kid.

Today, there is a huge shortage of people touching the dirt, and we are seeing the repercussions. I know there are many—thousands—of reasons why we are becoming the sickest species on the planet, but one of those reasons, and a very important one at that, is not taking the time to play in the dirt!

Back before beds were raised off the ground and all shoes had rubber soles, people would keep grounded naturally. They would sleep on the ground and walk with no shoes and socks, or with leather wrapped around their feet. In other words, they would play in the dirt. They had no idea doing this was incredibly important to their physical and mental well-being. It was just a normal part of life. We can say it was a lifestyle. Then came beds raised off the ground and rubber soles on shoes, but still almost all people grew some of their food; sometimes, all of it. Even though they weren't sleeping on the ground or walking almost barefoot, they were outside in the sun preparing the ground to plant. They also didn't know that it was important to stay grounded, to touch the earth often. They just did it; it was a lifestyle. One thing they did understand was that the earth was important to their overall well-being. As Hippocrates, the father of medicine, is quoted as saying:

"Illnesses do not come upon us out of the blue. They are developed from small daily sins against Nature. When enough sins have accumulated, illnesses will suddenly appear."

They understood that we need nature to be well. They also lived a lifestyle where they were in contact with the earth every day, some days for hours at a time.

Fast forward to today. As stated earlier, more than fifty percent of the world's population lives in cities. In many places, it is difficult just finding a plot of dirt. Many people are living a couple of stories above the ground in high-rise apartment buildings. We couldn't be farther from the earth in today's society. Sad, truly sad! Our health and well-being are paying the consequence.

Earthing!

Do a search on the Internet for the word "earthing" and see what results you get. You are probably going to be surprised that the English language now has a new word.

What in the world is earthing? Well, according to the book *Earthing: The Most Important Health Discovery Ever!*:

"Earthing is both a timeless practice and a modern discovery. It simply means living in contact with the Earth's natural surface charge."

It continues,

"In short, earthing restores and maintains the human body's most natural electrical state, which in turn promotes optimum health and functionality in daily life. The primordial natural energy emanating from the Earth is the ultimate anti-inflammatory and the ultimate anti-aging medicine."

So simple—let your bare feet touch the earth, but the health and lifestyle benefits are incalculable. By just having your feet in contract with the earth you are living a lifestyle that promotes healing, recuperation, building, and prevention. Wow!

What does placing our feet on the ground do that is so important to our health? One of the many things it does is decrease inflammation through free radical reduction.

Inflammation is the underlying cause of most chronic illnesses.

To understand the significance of taking off your shoes and socks and walking on earth, it is important to understand what free radicals are, what inflammation is, and what it is doing to modern societies and other societies following in their footsteps.

First, inflammation is very important in healing. Second, healing should be a temporary process. You get injured and your body heals. Once the healing is done, the inflammation should go away. That is not what is happening in today's world. There are many reasons why—from eating processed food to destructive self-talk. Today, we can say that most people are chronically inflamed.

Most people think of inflammation as an area of the body that is red, warm, swollen, and painful. These are known as the cardinal signs of inflammation. One sign that is not talked about as much, but is also present, can be a decrease in range of motion or loss of function. With chronic inflammation, we won't see the cardinal signs.

We usually won't see a red and swollen area that is warmer than the surrounding areas, as we see with an acute ankle sprain, for example. We will eventually experience pain with chronic inflammation, and that is what will usually move someone to seek help. But by that time, the inflammation has been present for a long time and has caused more damage than benefit.

When acute, or in other words, short-lived, the inflammation is one of the ways the body defends itself from bacteria, viruses, or any other type of bug our body sees as foreign. It also gets the healing process underway. The body's immune system sends in many different types of cells to take on the invader and clean up after trauma; some of these cells do it by releasing free radicals.

Our bodies not only release free radicals to fight back and eliminate the damaged tissue, but also normal essential metabolic processes create free radicals. When we digest the nutrient-dense food we are providing our ecosystems of cells, we form free radicals. When we contract our muscles as we lift a shovel-load of dirt, we form free radicals. Free radicals alone are not bad; they get the bad rap due to their overabundance because the lives we are living are completely incongruent with who we are. One of those incongruences is the disconnect from fertile soil in our lives.

What exactly are free radicals? A free radical is a molecule that has an unpaired electron. Free radicals are highly reactive because electrons like to be in a pair, and they will do anything to find that pair. The free radical can find the other much-needed electron to neutralize itself by fighting off bacteria or eliminating damaged tissue, or when there is an overabundance of free radicals, by stealing them from normal healthy tissue, causing damage to that tissue. With normal healthy tissue now damaged due to the overabundance of free radicals, the body sends the immune system to fix the damage, causing more inflammation and more free radicals. It turns into a vicious cycle of chronic inflammation.

"Inflammation is now believed to be the underlying cause of more than eighty chronic illnesses, and more than half of Americans suffer currently from one or more of them. Each year, millions die from these conditions." (3)

If just living forms free radicals, and living life in this modern world causes more free radicals, where can we go to get the electrons we need to form pairs and neutralize the overabundance of free radicals causing unnecessary inflammation and eventually unnecessary suffering, illness, and death?

Most people who have studied a little about the subject will say, "Antioxidants found in food." Yes, that is a great answer and another reason why it is so important to play in the dirt. We can grow food that is nutrient-dense that will provide antioxidants that will help neutralize some of the free radicals. There is even a better and easier answer to that question though. Take your shoes and socks off and go and stand on

(3) Ober, Clinton. *Earthing: The Most Important Health Discovery Ever!* Turner Publishing Company. 2010.

the earth; go walk on grass, the dirt, and the sand and receive the abundance of electrons our bodies need to neutralize free radicals.

The Earth's electrical surface charge is always negative, meaning that the surface is filled with free electrons just waiting to help neutralize free radicals.

Electrical engineers know that the surface of the Earth is pulsating with free electrons. And while medical scientists don't know that, they do know that the body is electrical in nature and that free radical molecules are on the lookout for electrons and are more than willing to take them from a stable molecule, a process that is at the core of inflammation, tissue destruction, and disease.

Soil is where the electron partner is found. Soil has a negative charge and with that electron or negative charge in the soil freely willing to partner with that electron in the free radical, we get a neutralized molecule that won't do us any harm.

There is a virtually limitless and continuously-renewed supply of electrons on the Earth's surface because of the core of the planet and all the lightning strikes that happen around the world. Maintaining contact with the ground allows our body to naturally receive and become charged with these electrons.

It's not just the fact that the surface of the Earth has a virtually limitless amount of electrons but,

"The sole (or plantar surface) of the foot is richly covered with some 1,300 nerve endings per square inch…That's more than found on any other part of the body of comparable size." (4)

We were created to touch the earth and, more importantly, with our bare feet! We could say that our feet are like the roots of a tree.

In addition, we are basically water and minerals, which makes us perfect conductors for those free electrons that are just waiting to neutralize the overabundance of free radicals that we have calming the inflammation in our bodies.

(4) Ober, Clinton. *Earthing: The Most Important Health Discovery Ever!* Turner Publishing Company. 2010.

Clint Ober said it perfectly:

"Earthing remedies an electrical instability and electron deficiency you never knew you had. It refills and recharges your body with something you never knew you were missing … or needed."

The earth literally grounds us.

By taking off your shoes and your socks and walking on the lush green grass, you decrease the cause of most illnesses: inflammation. This is because of the electrons found on the Earth's surface that neutralize free radicals. Incredible!

That should be reason enough to run outside right now, untie your shoes, throw them off along with your socks, and bathe in the healing reservoir called Planet Earth. But that truly is just the beginning.

All animals (including us) have an internal clock. Its job in its totality is to keep us at the top of our game. Since the invention of artificial light and the ability to use it to work and play all night long, our internal clock has become confused. It doesn't know when it is day and when it is actually night, making its job a lot more difficult, but it still tries.

This internal clock is called our circadian rhythm, and its main job is to get us ready for rest and work. Rest and work are both very important, and without a balance in both, we will eventually become ill. We have certain hormones that help us rest and others that help us work. When the sun goes down, usually around 9 p.m., depending on the season, an increase in the hormone called melatonin is seen in our ecosystem, helping us prepare to rest. This happens because when the eyes receive light from the sun, melatonin is inhibited, and when they don't receive the light from the sun, melatonin is produced, helping us prepare to rest.

When the sun is about to rise, around 6 a.m., we start to see an increase in cortisol, a hormone that gets us up and out working throughout the day.

The internal clock is very important, and if we live by its rules, it helps us maintain a healthy level of the proper hormones at the proper time. However, it isn't just the light from the sun that is received through the eyes that helps manage the sleep-wake cycle.

"The electrical potential present on the Earth's surface rises and falls according to the position of the sun. The intensity is more positive and energetic during the day, in support of your daily activities from wake up to shut down, and less positive and energetic during nighttime hours, promoting zzzzzzs. This daily high and low pattern sets in motion and orchestrates internal body mechanisms that regulate sleep-wake cycles, hormone production, and maintenance of health." (5)

As the Earth rotates, it helps maintain our natural internal clock through the electrical energy found on its surface. Electrical energy has also been found to work as a shield against electric fields that can disrupt the normal electric potentials of our bodies. This is because:

"[We] draw electrical energy through our feet in the form of free electrons fluctuating at many frequencies. These frequencies reset our biological clocks and

(5) Ober, Clinton. *Earthing: The Most Important Health Discovery Ever!* Turner Publishing Company. 2010.

provide the body with electrical energy. The electrons themselves flow into the body, equalizing and maintaining it at the electrical potential of the Earth. Just like standard electronic equipment that needs a stable ground to function well, so, too, the body needs stable grounding to also function well." (6)

Not too long ago, I felt the effects of an unstable standard electronic piece of equipment due to not being properly grounded. We had just bought a new washing machine, and the outlet we had it hooked up to outside was not properly grounded.

After the washer finishes with a load, what I usually do is just pull one piece of clothing out at a time and hang it on the clothesline. Many times, while I grab a piece of clothing, I will touch a part of the washer.

On one particular day, while I was outside hanging clothes on the line, I didn't have my shoes on. As I would grab a new piece of clothing to hang, I would slightly touch the washer and feel a sudden shock. It wasn't the shock you feel when you touch a door

(6) Ober, Clinton. *Earthing: The Most Important Health Discovery Ever!* Turner Publishing Company. 2010.

handle after walking on the carpet for a while, but a painful shock. I didn't think much of it until I touched the washing machine with a much larger portion of my body and received a pretty intense shock. I realized that something was not right. Our washing machine was not properly grounded and able to function properly due to that fact.

Eventually, we called an electrician. He stuck a metal rod in the ground and ran a grounding wire. He grounded the washing machine and also the refrigerator. Since then, I have never experienced that same shock touching the washer while barefoot, and I know that the washer and refrigerator are functioning properly.

We are the same. We also must ground ourselves to function properly and protect ourselves from other disruptive electric fields. This can only happen when we are physically touching the ground with bare hands or bare feet.

Clinton Ober says:

"Reconnecting to the Earth doesn't cure you of any disease or condition. What it does is reunite you with the natural electrical signals from the Earth that govern all organisms dwelling upon it. It restores your body's natural internal electrical stability and rhythms, which, in turn, promote normal functioning of body systems, including the cardiovascular, respiratory, digestive, and immune systems. It remedies an electron deficiency to reduce inflammation—the common cause of disease. It shifts the nervous system from a stress-dominated mode to one of calmness and better sleep. By reconnecting, you enable your body to return to its normal electrical state, better able to self-regulate and self-heal."

I couldn't have said it better. By playing in the dirt, we allow our systems that are electrical in nature to return to their normal and natural electrical state and function properly, thus enabling our ecosystem to regulate itself and if needed, heal itself. These systems include the nervous system, which controls all other systems, from the musculoskeletal and the cardiovascular all the way to the immune system.

Playing in the dirt neutralizes the overabundance of free radicals, calming inflammation, allowing us to thrive, and if needed, finally heal.

Playing in the dirt is an efficient way to protect ourselves from harm. It helps us maintain our electrically-powered ecosystem to keep it functioning in a proper and natural state. If our muscles are too tight, grounding will relax them; if our muscles are too relaxed, grounding will increase the tension to their natural state. Our bodies know best and combined with the beauty of nature and the healing power of the Earth, the possibilities of increased health and well-being are phenomenal.

Take time every day to ground yourself and reap the benefits of less physical, emotional, and spiritual pain—and really, of more health.

This is what the earth does for us. Yes, I have talked about various ways it will heal us, maintain us, and build us, but it all comes down to this. It restores us to our natural electrical and physiological state. It allows us as human beings, as an integral part of a marvelous ecosystem called Planet Earth, to be who we are supposed to be.

Playing in the dirt!

There are so many things we can and should learn from children. If we allow it, they can be our greatest examples of being present, in truly forgiving, in letting things go quickly, of understanding what is important, and in the importance of playtime. I could probably add quite a few more things.

Most adults have forgotten how to play. I say this from personal experience. I have made life too serious. As adults, we need to make time to play and that is why this book is titled *Playing in the Dirt*!

We need to take on the garden as if we are playing. It isn't a serious matter, and truly nothing in life should be taken too seriously.

Nature knows best; our job is just to play with her so she can work her miracles all around us and inside of us. When we become too serious about it, we begin to try and control nature, just like when we become serious about anything in life.

Life continues to teach me—and life is my best teacher, by the way. I have come to realize that control is a myth. The more we try to control, the more control we will lose. There is truly only one thing we can control, and that is how we act in or react to the internal or external environment we are currently placed in. If we learn to control the one thing we can—ourselves—we will always act and never react, and it will almost always be for the betterment of everybody and everything surrounding us.

As we let the control go and begin to play with nature, begin to play in the dirt, our lives will change—in many cases, drastically.

If you have lived incongruently with your ecosystem, you are now suffering from symptoms of some sort. By living the example set by the little ones, and just letting go and going outside and playing in the dirt, the changes you will see and feel will be dramatic.

If you believe you are living a healthy life, the changes may not be dramatic, but by playing in the dirt you will be healthier. You might not feel it now, but you will see and feel the difference as the years pass by. Your body will give you so much in return for just going out and playing with nature.

We have an important role in this beautiful ecosystem called Earth. If we act correctly, we can be a very fundamental part of making Earth a haven for health and healing. But if we continue on the path we are on, Earth will just become sicker and sicker; and the sicker that Earth is, the sicker we will become. We are now at a point where we need to make the decision now. How will we act?

Even though humans have destroyed so much of the fertile soil in the world, there is so much to be joyful about because as each one of us begins or continues to play with nature, as we play in the dirt, as we build soil, we can speed up the healing process of growing nutrient-dense soil: soil that is alive with billions of microorganisms in each handful. As we do this, we will speed the healing process of Planet Earth; and it will reward us, as we will also heal faster and feel better. We will have more energy, reach optimum weight, and aches and pains will disappear.

As we relinquish control and just decide to play in the dirt more often, we will reap the benefits of food that is true fuel for our ecosystems of cells.

After each meal, our cells will have a full tank of proper nutrition to heal, repair, or just increase overall health. We won't have to worry about what our bodies need because we will be certain that we are providing it. Our bodies will do all the rest. They will use what is needed at the exact moment in the exact amount. We will be giving our bodies proper nutrition. That can only come from what is grown in fertile soil without chemicals or from an animal that has eaten from a chemical-free fertile soil.

As we play in the dirt and build more, and more, fertile soil, we will experience the healing capacity of nature as the sun's rays reach our skin. As we run our hands through the microorganism-rich soil and allow those microorganisms to work with us, we will grow stronger and healthier together. It will bring us together as communities, where we will not just live but thrive.

As we play in the dirt, we can keep our bones and muscles strong by putting weight against them while moving more naturally and more often, keeping us as young as possible as the years pass.

As we play in the dirt, by getting outside and moving more naturally and more often, we can reduce the ever-increasing stresses that life seems to throw at us, allowing us to enjoy the moment and put aside those stresses of life. Also, by storing food that is grown in the garden to properly fuel ourselves and our families in those hard times that will eventually come, we will decrease the stress in an overall, very stressful moment in life.

If that isn't enough, the life in the soil can be considered a best friend, calming you down when you most need it. As the world becomes more and more of a hamster wheel that we run on each day, we find ourselves maxing out credit cards to just keep up, or at least to bring some pleasure into our lives over the weekend before we get right back on the hamster wheel. Just like the increase in serotonin levels we experience while hanging out talking to our friends or even petting our furry friends, by playing in the soil, the bacteria found there can increase serotonin levels to help us overcome the stresses of everyday life.

As you have read through the pages of this book, you probably noticed that I have had times in my life that have been very difficult. There were times where I thought there was no way out. These are difficult moments to live, and at least for me, even more difficult to put on paper so others can read about them. I have always considered myself more of a quiet person. I love community, I love learning from people, I love talking to people, but it isn't something I have to have, and I usually don't go looking for it.

I write about these things to show that it happens to all of us. There is not one person who goes through life without experiencing hard times. It is as normal as the rising sun. Unfortunately, many hard times are self-inflicted, but there are other hard times that will come no matter what. When those times arrive, it can feel like the rest of the world is doing just dandy. That isn't true; we all struggle at times to find who we truly are.

I continue to work and learn how to better control my internal environment and not allow what others say influence who I am. I continue to work and learn how to control my negative passions, like anger and envy. It is a lifelong process that becomes easier and easier. It is like anything that takes practice. When I first started playing basketball, the ball wouldn't even make it to the rim, but after shooting thousands of shots, the ball finds its way into the hoop more often.

Over the years, there have been times when I stopped playing basketball. Then when I returned to it, fewer shots were made due to lack of practice. Just like in basketball, if we want to become our best selves, we must practice every day.

Life is a lovely place to learn to be the best you. The hard times are where we will learn the most if we allow it.

While I was going through my hardest times, the garden helped me get through them. That is why this book is so important to me and why I bring it to you, the reader. It helped me feel physically healthy by helping me build a strong immune system throughout the years. Even though I was going through very difficult times, I have never really felt sick. I surprised the last doctor I talked to here in Argentina when she asked me if I had ever had an antibiotic. My answer was "no." She had a hard time believing it. Most people have used antibiotics on numerous occasions. By playing in the dirt and eating what fertile soil provides, my immune system has been able to strengthen itself. When I was at my lowest points, I was still able to feel physically healthy even though I was emotionally very sick.

Gardening has also helped me heal emotionally. It isn't enough that it helped build me up physically, but the garden was the first therapy that introduced me to being in the now, in a palpably and understandably way.

I still fear failure quite a bit, but the garden—even though it was just some flower pots and a small planter box at first—shows me that I can be here right now and not play back past events that haunt me or future events that scare me. It shows me that I can be right here right now and work, take one step forward, take one minute at a time, one hour at a time, one day at a time.

Playing in the dirt showed me how beautiful it is to be here right now. I have moved that into other aspects of my life, like drinking mate with my wife in the mornings. It helped me know the feeling of being in the zone, of having that altered state of consciousness that I so desperately needed. It continues to help me improve by making it easy to find gratitude in my life and being able to not only see it but feel it.

If the garden has done this for me, I know it can, and will, do the same for you.

If that wasn't enough, it has also kept me grounded, literally. As my body metabolizes, as it works and defends me, as I exercise, it naturally forms free radicals. As I took my shoes and socks off after a nice workout and planted my feet on the dirt or grass or sand, I was flooded with free electrons that neutralized those free radicals, calming the unhealthy effects that unchecked inflammation cause.

It has provided a literally invisible shield around me, blocking all odd frequencies. When I am outside playing in the dirt, I am in a natural and efficient electrical state, allowing my cells to send their electrical signals in a normal and healthy manner. It allows the cells, from neurons that control the nervous system to red blood cells that deliver life-giving oxygen to all the tissues of the body, to work as they were intended to work.

I am beyond excited to have been able to bring this to you, reader! It is something that not so long ago was pretty normal but unfortunately has become a rarity in today's society.

Some people still have their parents or grandparents that lived during World War II, when the famous "victory gardens" were promoted so the farmers could send their crops overseas to help the troops fighting in the war.

"[In] 1944, an estimated 20 million victory gardens produced roughly 8 million tons of food—which was the equivalent of more than 40 percent of all the fresh fruits and vegetables consumed in the United States." (7)

Not only that, but everybody was encouraged to have two hens for each person that lived in the house to provide much-needed protein. That wasn't that long ago. Almost 50 percent of all fruits and vegetables came from gardens planted in front yards, backyards, schools, and pretty much any empty lot that was available.

Either your parents, grandparents, or great grandparents at one time played in the dirt. Back then, it was for a different cause, but today it is just as important. Today, we need to play in the dirt for our own health and the health of our families and future

(7) https://www.history.com/news/americas- patriotic-victory-gardens

generations. We can't continue to treat nature the way we are treating her without negative consequences. The health of the earth and the health of the people in developed countries and those countries developing has continually gone down year after year. You now know one of the reasons why! How powerful! How liberating!

With this knowledge, you can now change the course of your health, the health of your family, and the health of the Earth. What makes this so wonderful is that it is simple. To start, all we need to do first is take off our shoes and socks more often. Walk more without shoes and touch the earth with our hands and bare feet more often.

Of course, that is only the start. To get the full benefit of nature, we need to play in the dirt. We need to compost all organic material and return it to the soil, continuing the cycle of life.

We need to plant seeds and nurture those plants as nature does, so we can then truly enjoy the fruits of our labor. That doesn't just mean enjoying the fruits and vegetables we will eventually harvest, but the time outside under the sun with family and friends. It's not just growing soil, but growing better and healthier together.

My hope with this book is to get you excited to return to your roots. To return to who you are is an integral part of the ecosystem called Planet Earth, with a very important part in keeping her stable and healthy. My hope is that you will start to heal this planet by composting, bringing back the soil life we so desperately need. My hope is that you plant a garden with your family; it can be as small as a couple of flower pots on your balcony, or if you have the room, a lot more. My hope is that you will take your shoes off and if you have kids that they'll take their shoes off, and everyone will walk barefoot on the grass and dirt.

If you do that, your family and you will benefit physically, emotionally, and spiritually.

As I always say to my kids as they enter school, "Make sure you don't have too much fun, but just enough!"

Let's do this! I would love to hear how you are playing in the dirt. This is a process where we are constantly learning. I have a private Facebook group where we continue to grow and learn. You are more than welcome to join it using the link www.pastosverdesfarm.com/extras where we talk about health, how to improve soil health and gardening among many other things. Courses on how to compost and grow some of your own food will soon be coming and those in the Facegroup group will be the first to see them! See you there!

As I stated at the beginning of this book, this is just the starting point! I hope the pages of this book have helped you understand why it is so important to return to nature. Your garden is your personal little edge of nature for your health and well-being.

Now how do you live this lifestyle? Join like-minded people that are on a mission to bring the garden and a connection to nature and earth into the forefront of their journey for greater health and well-being. I firmly believe enjoying the earth beneath us and the sun above us is the only way to achieve sustainable health as an individual and continuous sustainability for the human race as a whole!

Join us as wellness farmers today! Visit: https://pastosverdesfarm.com/subscription

I hope to talk to you personally very soon.

Check out my other book where you get a paradox-changing philosophy on how to reach your health and well-being potential.

Go to: _The 4 Pillars of Health: Your health and well-being made simple_.

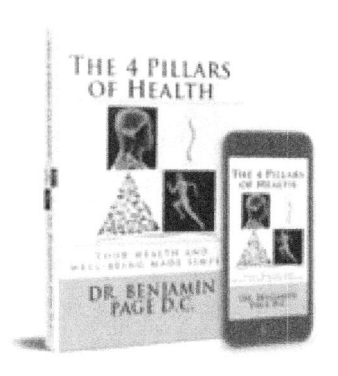

Acknowledgments

This was tough. It is not easy writing about dark times in one's life. But it is also beautiful to know that there are people out there who really want to help and who do help. First and foremost, I have to acknowledge my wife, Ruth, who puts up with me. Thanks for all that you do for me.

Thanks, Matías and Verena, my two awesome children, for being such great teachers and who motivate me to keep trying to be better.

Thanks to my parents for the way they raised me and how still, to this day, are always willing to help. No one is perfect, but I am truly grateful for the way they raised me. Thank you so much for helping me understand at a very young age the importance of health in a holistic way.

Thanks to Angela Frazier and Sue Peterson for helping with the editing of this book. Thanks for all the help and patience when I sent you messages with changes so often.

And, of course, thanks to you, the reader, for taking the time to read this creation of mine.

About the author

Benjamin Page is a chiropractic physician who works in the wellness paradigm. He helps his patients return to health through a holistic approach that includes care of the spine, nutrition through chemical-free food grown in fertile soils, adequate rest, sufficient movement, stretching, and the development of proper internal dialogue.

Benjamin is also the author of *The 4 Pillars of Health: Your Health and Well-being Made Simple*, and the creator of *The Wellness Farmer Podcast* and YouTube channel, where he shares his gardening journey in his little urban garden.

Made in the USA
Monee, IL
15 February 2023